Thyroid Disease

THE FACTS

R. I. S. BAYLISS, KCVO, MD, FRCP
*Consulting Physician and Endocrinologist,
Westminster Hospital, London; Consultant
Physician, King Edward VII's Hospital, London*

OXFORD
OXFORD UNIVERSITY PRESS
NEW YORK   TORONTO
1982

Oxford University Press, Walton Street, Oxford OX2 6DP

London Glasgow New York Toronto
Delhi Bombay Calcutta Madras Karachi
Kuala Lumpur Singapore Hong Kong Tokyo
Nairobi Dar es Salaam Cape Town
Melbourne Auckland

and associate companies in
Beirut Berlin Ibadan Mexico City Nicosia

British Library Cataloguing in Publication Data

Bayliss, R.I.S.
Thyroid disease. – (Oxford medical publications)
1. Thyroid gland – Diseases
I. Title
616.4'407   RC655
ISBN 0-19-261350-2

Library of Congress Cataloging in Publication Data
Bayliss, R.I.S.
Thyroid disease.
(Oxford medical publications)
Includes index.
1. Thyroid gland – Diseases.   I. Title.   II. Se-
ries. [DNLM: 1. Thyroid diseases – Popular works.
WK 200 B358t]
RC655.B39 1982   616.4'4   82-8082
ISBN 0-19-261350-2   AACR2

Set by Hope Services, Abingdon
Printed in Great Britain by R. Clay & Co.,
The Chaucer Press, Bungay, Suffolk.

Preface

The thyroid gland, which lies in the front of the neck, is one of the endocrine glands. Endocrine glands make chemical substances (hormones) which are passed into the bloodstream and influence the activity of cells in distant tissues and organs. In the case of the thyroid the action of its two hormones is to regulate the speed of activity of these distant cells in much the same way as the speed-control on a gramophone turn-table determines whether the record revolves at 78, 45, or $33\frac{1}{3}$ revolutions per minute. Increased production of thyroid hormones causes hyperthyroidism or thyrotoxicosis, and makes the cells of the body work too fast; too little production causes hypothyroidism, or, in its severest form, myxoedema in which the cells work sluggishly so that physical and mental activities are retarded.

Normally the thyroid gland can be felt in both men and women. Usually, however, it is invisible to the naked eye in men but may just be discernible in women. Any obvious enlargement is called a goitre, which simple means enlargement of the thyroid gland and which may be associated with normal, increased, or reduced hormone production. Indeed the size of the thyroid, or of any other endocrine gland for that matter, is a poor index of its hormonal output. Iodine is an essential constituent of the hormones made by the thyroid gland, and in regions of the world far distant from the sea (for example the Congo area, the Andes, and the Himalayas) goitre is common because iodine is deficient in the rain-water, in the soil, and hence in the food derived therefrom. The thyroid enlarges because it is striving to make its hormones without an essential ingredient — iodine: making bricks without straw.

Thyroid disease: the facts

Thyroid disease is common, although the prevalence varies considerably in different geographical areas. The incidence, for unexplained reasons, is always higher in women than men. The prevalence of hyperthyroidism is in women about 25 per 1000 population in the United Kingdom, and in men about 2 per 1000. Underactivity of the thyroid gland (hypothyroidism) of varying intensity has a prevalence of the order of 15 women per 1000 and of men only 1 per 1000. Obvious goitres occur in about 7 per cent of the population in non-iodine-deficient areas and are four times more common in women than men.

It is hoped that this book will be of help to people with thyroid disease. I use the word 'people' rather than 'patients' because many, despite requiring treatment over many years, may not feel ill. Doctors are well aware that in most diseases the greater the patients' understanding of their condition, the fewer are their fears and the better is the acceptance and outcome of treatment. Such is certainly the case in disorders of the thyroid gland.

The workings of the thyroid gland, its manufacture of hormones, and its control are complex. So also are the disorders that lead to overactivity or underactivity of the gland. I have tried to resist the temptation to expand too fully on matters which are more the concern of biochemists, epidemiologists, and those of us in the clinical field who endeavour to advance the frontiers of knowledge. Simplification may be helpful to patients, to junior medical students, nurses, and other paramedical professionals; it may not appeal to expert thyroidologists. But this is a book for understanding and rightly has to stand alongside other titles in this distinguished and I believe useful series.

This book owes much to those who have taught me most about thyroid disorders, without their being held responsible for my views: to former teachers and colleagues such as Dr Harold Gardiner-Hill, Professor Russell Fraser, Professor Noel Maclagan, Professor John Hobbs, Dr Joan Zilva, and

Preface

Professor Reginald Hall in England, and Professors Sidney
Werner and Henry Aranow in New York; to the patients
from many lands who unquestionably have taught me most
and whom it has been my happy privilege to treat or supervise;
and not least to my non-medical wife who has read the text
and helped me render it comprehensible.

I am most grateful to Mr Keith Duguid, Head of the
Department of Medical Illustration at Westminster Hospital,
for the photographic work and to Dr C.R. Bayliss for the
illustrations used in Plate 4.

London   R.I.S.B.
January 1982

Contents

1

Where and what is the thyroid gland?

Normally the thyroid gland is located in the front of the neck just below the Adam's apple (thyroid cartilage). It consists of two lobes, each about the size and shape of half a large plum cut vertically. These lobes lie to the right and left of the mid-line, on either side of the windpipe (trachea), and are connected by a small bridge of thyroid tissue (the isthmus) which runs across the front of the trachea (Fig. 1).

In men the normal gland is seldom sufficiently large to be visible, but in many women it is just discernible to the naked eye, particularly when the chin is lifted up. When visible the gland can be seen to move up and down in the neck when the patient swallows. Normally in both sexes the two lobes can be felt by the doctor's examining fingers. The healthy gland is smooth and firm – not nodular or hard. In some patients it may extend downwards to lie wholly or in part behind the upper part of the breastbone (a retrosternal thyroid gland).

In the fetus the thyroid gland develops in the region of the root of the tongue. Before birth the gland normally descends down the neck to occupy its usual position. The path of this descent is marked by a small rudimentary cord – the thyroglossal duct – which sometimes persists and in adult life can become filled with fluid. This causes a small cyst in the mid-line of the neck vertically above the thyroid gland. A thyroglossal cyst is of no clinical consequence unless it is unsightly, but it may be confused with a cyst or nodule in the thyroid gland itself. The main point of distinction is that a thyroglossal cyst usually moves vertically upwards in the neck when the tongue is protruded by the patient.

Occasionally the thyroglossal duct persists as the pyramidal lobe of the thyroid gland. This is an extra lobe of the thyroid

1

Thyroid disease: the facts

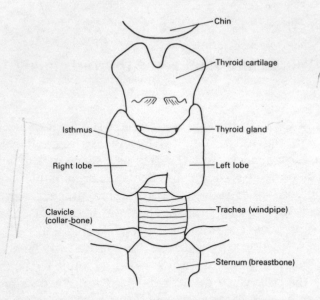

Fig. 1. The anatomy of the thyroid gland.

gland which is an upward extension of the isthmus: it may lie in the mid-line or extend upwards for 1–2 inches lying on either side of the larynx.

In some babies the thyroid does not descend properly and remains imperfectly developed in its embryonic position near the root of the tongue. Such an ectopically placed thyroid gland seldom functions properly, and maldescent or mal-development is a common cause of thyroid deficiency (cretinism) in new-born babies (Chapter 7).

Goitre is the term used to describe an enlarged thyroid gland. This enlargement may be very slight or more obvious and sometimes may even be quite massive. Enlargement of the thyroid implies some abnormality but in many instances this is not a serious or indeed significant matter. There are many causes of goitre, and the size of the gland is a very poor index of its activity or secretory function. Thus a large gland may be underactive, and a small goitre or normal sized gland may be associated with overactivity.

Where and what is the thyroid gland?

Secretory function

The thyroid is an endocrine gland. Thus, like other endocrine glands (the pituitary gland, the pancreas, the ovaries in women and the testes in men, the adrenal glands, and the parathyroid glands), the thyroid manufactures certain chemical substances (hormones) that are secreted into the bloodstream and induce an effect on cells and tissues elsewhere in the body.

The thyroid makes two hormones — thyroxine, which because this chemical compound contains four iodine atoms is often called T_4, and triiodothyronine which contains three iodine atoms and for brevity is called T_3. Both are secreted into the bloodstream and are carried round the body. In the distant peripheral tissues the thyroxine (T_4) is converted to triiodothyronine (T_3) and it is the T_3 that exerts its influence on all body cells. It is not entirely clear why the thyroid produces two hormones. The probable explanation is that T_3 has a relatively immediate effect on the cells of the body whereas the influence of T_4 is slower because it has first to be converted to T_3. Thus the metabolic activity of cells is subject to control by a quick acting and a more slowly acting hormone.

Both hormones are transported in the circulation loosely attached to certain proteins in the blood. When bound to these carrier proteins T_4 and T_3 are biologically inactive; only when the thyroxine and triiodothyronine are freed from their protein binding and are present in the water of the blood are they active. This is of some importance when it comes to laboratory tests for measuring the blood level of T_4 and T_3 because current methods largely measure the protein-bound hormones.

The manufacture of thyroid hormones

The two thyroid hormones — thyroxine (T_4) and triiodothyronine (T_3) — are formed by the cells in the thyroid gland.

3

Thyroid disease: the facts

An essential ingredient is iodine and this is preferentially extracted from the bloodstream by the thyroid cells. Thus iodine must be available in the body. It is normally provided by the food we eat and comes from the water and soil in which our vegetables are grown. The iodine is derived from the rain that falls on the earth, and this in turn comes from the water vapourized from the sea to form the rain. Areas of the world far removed from rain derived from sea-water (the Congo area in Africa, the Andes in South America, the Himalayas in the Indian subcontinent, Switzerland in Central Europe, the Great Lakes area in the USA, and certain areas in other land masses — Spain and Iran) are deficient in iodine. People living in such areas have difficulty in making thyroid hormones because they are deprived of iodine (Chapter 7), unless public-health steps are taken to supplement their dietary iodine intake.

Within the cells of the thyroid gland, the iodine is amalgamated by a number of complicated chemical steps with other substances to form T_4 and T_3. These hormones are then stored within the cells of the thyroid loosely coupled with a protein in the form of thyroglobulin. The rate with which iodine is extracted from the bloodstream and taken into the thyroid cells is regulated by the thyroid-stimulating hormone (see below) secreted by the pituitary gland. This hormone also controls the rate at which T_4 and T_3, stored as thyroglobulin in the thyroid cells, are released from storage and secreted into the bloodstream.

Biological effect

What do the thyroid hormones do? In many respects they can be likened in their action to the speed control on a gramophone. They regulate the metabolic activity of all body cells and tissues. Too little thyroid hormone means that the body cells work at too slow a rate. The result is much the same as playing a 45 r.p.m. record at $33\frac{1}{3}$ r.p.m.; it is slowed and

4

Where and what is the thyroid gland?

lugubrious. By contrast too much hormone induces the cells to work too fast. The $33\frac{1}{3}$ r.p.m. record is played at 45 r.p.m. and the result is a 'chipmunk' effect. More precise clinical details of thyroid overactivity (hyperthyroidism) and underactivity (hypothyroidism) are given in Chapters 4 and 7.

Although the two thyroid hormones influence the proper working of all body cells, their effect is particularly evident in certain functions. For example growth and development, both physical and mental, depend upon the presence of an adequate amount of thyroxine. Without thyroxine a tadpole will not metamorphose into a frog, and without thyroxine a new-born baby will not grow properly nor will its brain develop properly. Thyroxine regulates the rate of oxygen consumption, which is another way of saying it controls the speed of activity of body cells. It influences how the body utilizes food by influencing the metabolism of sugar, protein, and fat. In thyroid deficiency, for instance, the level of a particular fat, cholesterol, often increases in the bloodstream. This results in arteries becoming clogged up because cholesterol is deposited in the inner wall of the blood-vessels and their lumen is narrowed.

Control of thyroid gland function

How is the thyroid gland controlled? What determines the amount of T_4 and T_3 secreted into the bloodstream? This is complex but the fundamental control mechanism is relatively simple to understand. It can be likened to the thermostatic control of the temperature in a house by the effect that the thermostat in the hall or sitting room has on the gas or oil-fired furnace.

The secretory activity of the thyroid gland is regulated by the pituitary gland's secretion of thyroid-stimulating hormone (TSH or thyrotrophin). The pituitary gland is the size of a grape and lies at the base of the brain. It secretes many different hormones including the thyroid-stimulating hormone (TSH). This hormone passes into the bloodstream and activates the thyroid gland to secrete more T_4 and T_3. As a result of this stimulation of the thyroid cells, the level of T_4 and T_3 in the bloodstream rises; the pituitary cells that secrete TSH sense this and the output of thyroid-stimulating hormone is reduced (Fig. 2). This feed-back control

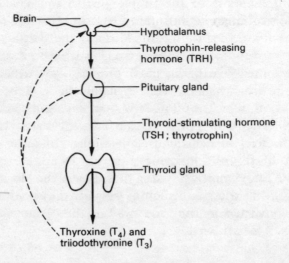

Fig. 2. Mechanisms controlling the secretion by the thyroid gland of thyroxine (T_4) and triiodothyronine (T_3). As the levels of T_4 and T_3 rise in the bloodstream, the secretion of thyrotrophin releasing hormone (TRH) from the hypothalamus and of thyroid-stimulating hormone (TSH) from the pituitary is reduced or switched off (feedback control mechanism). As the levels of T_4 and T_3 fall, the hypothalamus secretes more TRH and the pituitary gland more TSH so that activity of the thyroid gland is increased.

is similar to the thermostat that senses when the temperature in the house has risen to the required degree and then turns off the furnace so that heat production is stopped or reduced. Conversely when the blood levels of T_4 and T_3 fall below a certain point, the TSH-secreting cells of the pituitary gland recognize this, and produce more thyroid-stimulating hormone: this activates the thyroid cells to increase their output

Where and what is the thyroid gland?

of T_4 and T_3 just as when the room temperature falls below a certain point the thermostat activates the furnace to produce more heat.

The control mechanism is made more delicate (and more complex) by the fact that the sensitivity of the pituitary gland (equivalent to the setting of the thermostat) is determined by the hypothalamus. This is another endocrine gland located in the brain close to the pituitary. The hypothalamus also secretes a number of hormones that control the sensitivity and activity of the pituitary gland. The hypothalamic chemical that influences the TSH-secreting cells of the pituitary is the thyrotrophin-releasing hormone (TRH). The output of TRH from the hypothalamic cells is regulated — turned on and off — by the levels of T_4 and T_3 in the bloodstream in the same way as the TSH-secreting cells of the pituitary are (Fig. 2). The hypothalamus is however more complex than the pituitary gland. It can be likened to a micro-chip computer. Apart from T_4 and T_3, it is sensitive to many less well-defined influences, such as possibly the weather, season, and external temperature and the patient's 'temperament'.

7

2

Disorders of the thyroid gland

Some diseases are specific or particular to the thyroid gland and do not, indeed cannot, occur elsewhere in the body. For example overactivity of the gland and underactivity are, in the symptoms produced, diseases peculiar to the thyroid. Certain other disorders such as acute or subacute inflammation (thyroiditis) and cancer are not so specific to the thyroid because inflammation or malignant change occurs in other organs. Nevertheless the clinical picture of inflammation or cancer of the thyroid gland will be strongly coloured by the fact that the disease process is located in this organ.

Simple goitre

Any enlargement of the thyroid gland constitutes a goitre, which may be small or large. The qualifying adjective 'simple' does not imply that the mechanism causing this enlargement is simple to explain; indeed often it is complex. In this context 'simple' means that the goitre is not associated with any detectable increase or decrease in thyroid secretory activity. The patient does not have hyperthyroidism or hypothyroidism. A normal amount of thyroid hormones is being produced: the blood levels of T_4 and T_3 are within the normal range. The patient is therefore euthyroid, not hyperthyroid or hypothyroid. Thus the goitre is 'simple' from the secretory point of view, and in addition it is benign as opposed to being cancerous or malignant.

The causes of goitre in a euthyroid subject are discussed in detail in Chapter 8, but in many instances it is difficult to determine the cause of thyroid enlargement. Some enlargement of the gland is so common in women at the time of

8

puberty, during pregnancy, and during the menopause, that this can be looked upon as normal or physiological. Enlargement of the thyroid gland is also common, more so in women than men, in areas of the world where there is deficiency of iodine in the diet. A goitre may also develop, perhaps surprisingly, in people who take iodine-containing medicines — usually proprietary cough mixtures — and other drugs over a prolonged period of time. Simple goitres are not painful. If large they may be cosmetically unsightly but small goitres used to be considered attractive in women and many of the portraits by the prolific Dutch court painter Lely (1618–80) show this. Only rarely is a simple goitre of sufficient size to press on the windpipe and cause difficulty in breathing, or to interfere with swallowing.

Hypothyroidism

Underactivity of the thyroid gland is considered more fully in Chapter 7. It may occur in infancy due to inadequate development or maldescent of the thyroid gland before the baby is born (p. 73). Later in life hypothyroidism may be the consequence of removal of too much thyroid tissue during surgical treatment of hyperthyroidism or of destruction of too much thyroid tissue by radio-iodine treatment of hyperthyroidism (Chapter 4).

Autoimmune destruction of the thyroid. The commonest 'natural' cause of hypothyroidism is autoimmune chronic thyroiditis, also called Hashimoto's thyroiditis. Some knowledge of autoimmune processes is essential to the understanding of two common thyroid disorders — hypothyroidism, which left untreated progresses to its severest form, namely myxoedema, and hyperthyroidism as occurs in Graves' disease (so called after the Dublin physician who described the condition in 1832).
Autoimmune disorders are an extension of the normal

bodily defence mechanisms against infection. Certain white corpuscles in the blood (lymphocytes) recognize as 'foreign' micro-organisms (bacteria or viruses) which enter the body. The situation is analagous to soldiers becoming aware that foreign enemy troops have penetrated their defences. Just as the soldiers round up the enemy troops and kill or try to kill them, so the lymphocytes form chemical substances called antibodies that kill off the invading micro-organisms. Foreign proteins of any sort are looked upon as invaders by the lymphocytes and antibodies are formed by these white cells to immobilize and kill the enemy. This is why there are problems when an organ like the kidney, which is essentially made of protein, is transplanted from one person to another. The lymphocytes of the recipient look upon the donated kidney as 'foreign', which it is; they attack it and, without special intervention by the doctor, would destroy it. This rejection by the recipient is one of the major problems in transplanting kidneys, hearts, and other organs. If the donated kidney comes from somebody totally unrelated to the recipient and if the donor has a totally different blood group from that of the recipient, the lymphocytes immediately spot the donated kidney as foreign and attack it fiercely. If on the other hand the donated kidney comes from an identical twin of the recipient, the lymphocytes in the recipient may hardly recognize the kidney as an enemy and the extent of rejection is very much less. Hence the greater success of a kidney transplant from an identical twin or a close relative.

In autoimmune disorders, for reasons which we do not yet fully understand, the lymphocytes get the mistaken idea that some tissue or organ in the body is 'foreign'. It is like one group of soldiers getting wrong intelligence and thinking that the troops serving alongside them are the enemy. In the case of thyroid autoimmune disorders, the lymphocytes react against the cells or constituents of the cells of the thyroid gland. Antibodies are formed in the bloodstream and the strength of concentration of these autoantibodies can be measured. In the case of Hashimoto's thyroiditis (named after the Japanese doctor who described the microscopic appearance of the thyroid gland in this condition) the antibodies promote the destruction of the thyroid cells. This is often a slow process occurring over many years.

Hyperthyroidism

The commonest form of hyperthyroidism is that produced by Graves' disease, in which the whole of the thyroid gland becomes overactive. This increased activity is due to the formation of antibodies by lymphocytes, many of which may be found interspersed between the thyroid cells. In contrast to Hashimoto's disease, the antibodies in Graves' disease stimulate the cells of the thyroid to secrete increased amounts of T_4 and T_3. In other words these antibodies mimic the action of thyroid-stimulating hormone. Less commonly thyrotoxicosis is caused by a small nodule of cells in the thyroid that secretes too much hormone, a so-called toxic nodule (see Chapter 4).

Thyroiditis

Occasionally the thyroid gland becomes infected with microorganisms such as streptococci or the tubercle bacillus. More commonly it is attacked by a virus. This subacute thyroiditis (also called de Quervain's thyroiditis after a Swiss physician who first described it) may be caused by many different viruses including that which causes mumps. The condition is called subacute because the degree of discomfort in the neck due to inflammation of the thyroid gland is relatively slight but tends to persist, if untreated, for several weeks. The gland is tender to the touch and swallowing may be painful (Chapter 6).

Cancer

Among the disorders of the thyroid gland cancer is rare, and among malignant growths in the body as a whole it is even rarer. Most thyroid cancers are well differentiated; this means that the cells which make up the cancer continue to look, under the microscope, like relatively normal thyroid cells. These malignant cells do not usually multiply rapidly and hence the tumour does not grow fast. Often the cancerous cells retain many of the properties of normal thyroid cells: for instance they may remain responsive to the action of thyroid-stimulating hormone and they may continue to extract iodine from the bloodstream. This means that in addition to surgical removal of the growth, which is the corner-stone of treatment, any remaining malignant cells can be eliminated by radio-iodine treatment (see Chapter 9). Provided the condition is diagnosed early, the treatment of a differentiated thyroid cancer is usually very successful.

3

Investigation of thyroid disorders

The investigations useful in providing more information as to the nature of a disorder of the thyroid gland can be divided into two main categories.

First there are those tests that are used to determine the hormone secretory function of the gland and which therefore tell us whether the thyroid is producing the correct amount or too little or too much of the thyroid hormones.

Secondly there are tests that may give information as to what is wrong with the thyroid, and will answer such questions as 'why is the gland enlarged?', 'what is the nature of a circumscribed lump in one part of the gland; is it a simple benign lump or is it malignant?', 'why has this gland become underactive and is now secreting too little T_4 and T_3?'

Tests of thyroid secretory function

Over the years many different techniques have been used to determine whether the thyroid gland is making too much or too little hormone. In the old days the methods were often imprecise and indirect. Because it was not then technically feasible to measure T_4 and T_3, such indirect tests as the *basal metabolic rate* (BMR) were used. In this the patient's consumption of oxygen was measured over a given time; the hyperthyroid patient with an increased metabolic rate used more oxygen from the inspired air than a hypothyroid patient with a decreased metabolic rate. Useful as it was in those days, the technique was imprecise because the consumption of oxygen was influenced by additional factors other than the amount of thyroid hormone secreted.

The *cholesterol* level is also influenced by the amount of

13

thyroid hormone secreted. Cholesterol is a particular type of fat that circulates in the bloodstream. The level is raised in hypothyroidism and tends to be low in hyperthyroidism but the cholesterol is influenced by many other factors, and variations from normal in thyroid disease may occur only when the degree of disordered thyroid secretory function is extreme and of long standing.

The *tendon reflexes*, such as the well-known knee-cap reflex when the tendon just below the patella is tapped with a hammer, is in its speed of reaction influenced by the level of thyroid hormones. In practice the ankle reflex, judged by tapping on the Achilles tendon at the back of the lower leg, is usually used to assess thyroid function. The reflex is slowed in hypothyroidism and unduly rapid in hyperthyroidism. Electronic apparatus can be used to time the ankle reflex and the result is expressed in thousandths of a second. This test, too, is influenced by factors other than the level of thyroid hormones circulating in the bloodstream, and although it can be useful in measuring the patient's response to treatment it is of limited value in the primary diagnosis of hyperthyroidism or hypothyroidism.

The *uptake of radio-iodine* was more recently used as an index of thyroid function. This test is based on the fact that the uptake of iodine, or one of its radioactive isotopes, by the gland is increased in hyperthyroidism when the production of excess thyroid hormone requires more iodine to make the T_4 and T_3. Conversely less iodine, or radioactive iodine, is taken up when the gland is manufacturing less than normal amounts of the thyroid hormones.

The uptake of radio-iodine is measured by giving the patient by mouth or by intravenous injection a radioactive iodine isotope and measuring with a Geiger–Muller counter placed over the thyroid gland the amount of the radio-iodine that enters the gland at 2–6 hours in patients suspected of hyperthyroidism and at 24–48 hours in those suspected of hypothyroidism.

14

Investigation of thyroid disorders

This is, however, an indirect method of assessing the production of T_4 and T_3. The situation is similar to that in a car factory, in which iodine is akin to the steel going into the factory. It could be argued that the more raw material (in this case steel) that goes into the factory the more cars are coming out at the other end. Over a prolonged period of time this would probably be true, but in the short term all sorts of fallacies may arise. The factory might be stockpiling steel and holding it in store without increasing car production. The factory might be making the usual number of cars but storing them in the factory and not releasing them for sale. Similarly with iodine, an increase in uptake may indicate stockpiling perhaps because the thyroid gland has for a time been starved of iodine. Thus increased uptake cannot invariably be equated with increased secretion of T_4 and T_3. The uptake of radio-iodine is reduced when there is hypothyroidism due to destruction of the gland from, for example, autoimmune processes such as occurs in Hashimoto's thyroiditis (Chapter 6). Even though the thyroid may be capable of normal hormone production, the uptake of radio-iodine will be suppressed if the patient is taking T_4 or T_3 by mouth: such medication will suppress the secretion of TSH from the patient's pituitary gland and this will put the thyroid gland into a resting inactive state. Perhaps the most instructive example of the possibly misleading result obtained by radio-iodine uptake in relation to secretory activity is given by thyroiditis due to a virus infection (Chapter 5). In this condition the thyroid cells are disorganized by the inflammation. They cannot work properly and hence the uptake of iodine is virtually zero. However the inflammatory process causes pre-formed T_4 and T_3 stored in the thyroglobulin colloid to be released into the circulation so that the patient exhibits the symptoms and signs of hyperthyroidism.

Various different isotopes of iodine are used for these studies. ^{131}I is most often given, but sometimes ^{123}I or ^{132}I are used because they have a shorter life, which means they decay more rapidly than ^{131}I and hence cause less general irradiation to the patient: they are preferred for studies in children and whenever repeated tests have to be made. Patients given these isotopes in the trace amounts needed to assess thyroid uptake can be confidently reassured that the irradiation hazard is negligible. Another isotope, technetium, ^{99m}Tc, is nowadays for reasons of technical convenience often used in place of iodine radio-isotopes, but has to be administered intravenously. Technetium is taken up by the thyroid cells in the same way as iodine is trapped but it is not incorporated by the complex chemical steps in the manufacture of T_4 and T_3. This and radio-iodine now find their main use in determining what is wrong with the thyroid rather than in assessing its secretory function. The use of isotopes in scanning is discussed on p. 26.

For a decade (1960–70) the *protein-bound iodine* (PBI) level in the bloodstream was used as an index of thyroid secretory activity. This technique assumed that the amount of iodine bound to protein in the bloodstream was an index of the amount of T_4 and T_3 present. Admittedly both contain iodine and are bound to protein, but the PBI also measures non-hormonal iodine attached to protein, and this is increased for months or even years, for example, after special X-rays that use iodine-containing drugs to determine the radiological function and anatomy of the kidneys or the gall-bladder. It is also increased if the patient has taken iodine-containing medicines. Furthermore the rather difficult chemical analysis can be vitiated if the laboratory in which it is performed becomes contaminated with iodine which can happen if somebody, perhaps a cleaner, goes in sucking an iodized cough lozenge.

Fortunately modern techniques allow us to measure accurately and specifically the levels of thyroxine (T_4) and triiodothyronine (T_3) in the bloodstream. The methods now used (radioimmune assay) have made for great accuracy in the assessment of thyroid hormone secretion.

16

Investigation of thyroid disorders

Serum thyroxine (T_4) level. This is measured in a small sample of blood obtained from a vein. The result can be obtained in about 48 hours. The amount of hormone present may be expressed in terms of the weight of T_4 per 100 ml of blood or in terms of the number of molecules of T_4 per litre. Although the normal range will always be within the same order of magnitude, it will differ slightly from one laboratory to another depending on the exact chemicals (reagents) used and the population of 'healthy' people from whose results the normal range has been determined. In most instances of hyperthyroidism the result of the T_4 estimation is unequivocally above this normal range, and in patients with hypothyroidism it is below it.

The main snag about measuring the total serum T_4 level is that the method used measures the amount of thyroxine bound to carrier-protein (see Chapter 1). Strictly speaking it is the 0.015 per cent or thereabouts of the thyroxine which is unbound to protein and floating free in the water of the blood that determines the patient's thyroid status. Thus the total (protein-bound and much smaller amount of free) thyroxine is measured, and hence the result is influenced by two factors — the amount of thyroxine present and the amout of carrier-protein.

Under certain circumstances, for example in pregnancy, or when taking oestrogens, or the contraceptive pill, or certain other drugs, the amount of carrier protein is increased. This increases the total T_4 level but does not make the subject hyperthyroid because the free non-protein-bound thyroxine remains normal. Some drugs as aspirin and several others (see Table 1) may occupy the binding sites on the carrier-protein normally reserved for thyroxine. These drugs will tend to lower the T_4 level by reducing the protein-bound thyroxine but they will not make the patient clinically hypothyroid because the free non-protein-bound thyroxine will remain normal.

Because of these variations in the thyroxine-binding protein level or of the binding sites, which are only occasionally of

17

Table 1 *Causes of altered thyroxine-binding proteins (TBP) or receptor sites on the carrier proteins*

Increased TBP
  Pregnancy
  Oestrogen therapy
  Oral contraceptive pill
  Clofibrate (Atromid-S) therapy
  Phenothiazine (e.g. chlorpromazine, Largactil) therapy
  Myxoedema
  Hereditary increased TBP

Decreased TBP or reduced binding sites
  Kidney disease or other conditions causing low plasma proteins
  Thyrotoxicosis
  Acromegaly
  Cushing's syndrome (hyperadrenocorticism)
  Hereditary low or absent TBP
  Anabolic, androgenic, or corticosteroid therapy
  Fenclofenac (Flenac) therapy
  Phenylbutazone (Butazolidine, Butacote) therapy
  Phenytoin (Epanutin, Dilantin) therapy
  Salicylate (e.g. aspirin) therapy

major practical importance, various corrective procedures may be used to assess the level of the carrier-proteins and to make appropriate allowance for these proteins or their binding sites being increased or decreased.

Thyroxine-binding globulin. One way is to measure the exact amount of thyroxine-binding globulin (TBG) that is present in the patient's blood. This is the most important and significant of the several thyroxine-binding proteins in the bloodstream but this technique is not widely available, and has certain limitations. An alternative procedure is to measure the binding sites on the carrier-proteins that are unoccupied by thyroxine. This is done in the so-called resin uptake test in which the unoccupied binding sites are measured with radioactive T_3 rather than T_4, because the affinity of the binding sites is much stronger for T_4 than T_3 which does not displace the thyroxine molecules already attached to the proteins (Fig. 3).

Investigation of thyroid disorders

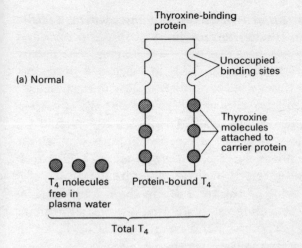

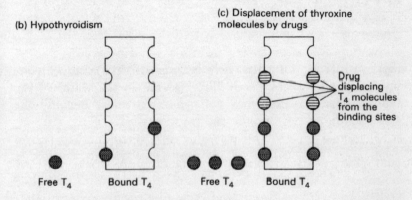

Fig. 3. The binding of thyroxine (T_4) by carrier-proteins in the blood-stream. (a) Normal. Molecules of T_4 are attached to binding sites on the thyroxine-binding protein. There are some unoccupied binding sites, the number of which can be measured by the T_3 resin test (see text). The subject's thyroid status is determined by the T_4 molecules floating free in the water of the blood and amount to only 0.015 per cent of the total thyroxine (bound and unbound). (b) Hypothyroidism. There is a reduced amount of thyroxine, both protein-bound and free. More of the binding sites on the carrier protein are unoccupied. (c) Displacement by a drug (see text) of T_4 molecules from their binding sites on the carrier-protein. The total amount of thyroxine is reduced, but the patient remains euthyroid because the free thyroxine remains normal.

19

T_3 resin binding test. There can be few tests which, because of nomenclature, have caused more confusion amongst patients and also amongst doctors than this one! The precise technique need not detain us. It is in essence a procedure designed to determine whether a high or low thyroxine level is solely the consequence of a change in the amount of carrier-protein or a change in the available sites on the protein for carrying thyroxine. It is *not* a measure in any way of the second thyroid hormone, triiodothyronine (T_3). By itself the T_3 resin-binding test is of little value; its main use is for 'correcting' the value of the total serum thyroxine, upwards or downwards, depending upon whether the carrier-proteins or their binding sites are decreased or increased. This correction is incorporated in the 'free thyroxine index'.

Free thyroxine index. This is not really a test in its own right. It is a mathematical calculation derived from the total serum thyroxine level and the T_3 resin-binding test. It makes allowance for alterations, upwards or downwards, in the carrier-proteins and reflects the amount of thyroxine which is unattached to protein and floating free in the water of the blood. This is really what one wants to know because the free thyroxine determines the thyroid status of the patient. New techniques are already being developed for widespread application that will it is hoped measure the free thyroxine directly without any interference from the thyroxine-binding proteins.

Serum triiodothyronine (T_3) level. This is a measure of the serum protein-bound concentration of the second thyroid hormone. Usually the T_3 level moves in parallel with the T_4 level because one-third of the T_3 is secreted by the thyroid gland and two-thirds is derived in peripheral tissues from the conversion of T_4 to T_3. Only under rare circumstances is it necessary to measure the T_3 when the T_4 is being determined. However in a small proportion of hyperthyroid patients, particularly in the early phases of the disease or in patients

Investigation of thyroid disorders

who live in relatively iodine-deficient parts of the world, the T_3 is increased whereas the T_4 level remains in the normal range or only later becomes elevated. Thus occasionally one encounters a patient who has symptoms and signs highly suspicious of hyperthyroidism but yet the T_4 level is normal. In such rare instances the T_3 should be measured and this may confirm that the patient is indeed thyrotoxic. This condition is known as T_3 toxicosis (Chapter 4).

The T_3 level is also of value in monitoring the correct dosage of triiodothyronine in those hypothyroid patients who are treated with this compound rather than with thyroxine. Such patients will continue to have low T_4 serum levels although they may be euthyroid or even hyperthyroid depending on the amount of triiodothyronine they are taking.

Thyroid-stimulating hormone (TSH) level. The TSH level is normally quite low. In hyperthyroidism caused by auto-antibodies (p. 11) that are stimulating the gland to secrete excess T_4 and T_3, the pituitary and hypothalamus are switched off so that less TSH is produced (Fig. 2). The method used for measuring TSH is not good for distinguishing between the normal low levels in a euthyroid patient from the even lower levels found in a hyperthyroid patient; and here this test is unhelpful.

It is, however, of great help in confirming hypothyroidism. When a patient is grossly hypothyroid the T_4 level is un-equivocally below the normal range. In an attempt to activate the failing gland the hypothalamus increases its secretion of thyrotrophin-releasing hormone (Fig. 2) and the pituitary secretes increased amounts of TSH. The TSH level is raised and it is increased in proportion to the decrease in the serum T_4 level. Thus markedly low T_4 levels are associated with greatly increased TSH levels. When the degree of hypo-thyroidism is more marginal and the T_4 level is at or just below the normal range, the TSH level will be increased to a lesser degree, but this is of great help in confirming the

21

diagnosis. Indeed experience has shown that in failure of the thyroid gland, the TSH level is the most sensitive test for detecting this defect.

Table 2 *A summary of some common results of tests of thyroid secretory function and their significance*

Total T_4 level	Total T_3 level	TSH level	Significance
High	High	Normal	Hyperthyroidism or excess treatment with T_4 or increased TBP*
Normal	High	Normal	Hyperthyroidism (T_3 toxicosis)
Low	Normal or high	Normal	Treatment with T_3 (or endemic goitre)
Low	Normal or high	High	Subclinical or mild thyroid failure
Normal	Normal	High	Subclinical or mild thyroid failure
Normal	Normal	Normal	Normal (or hypothyroidism adequately treated with T_4)
Normal	Low	Normal	Generalized ill-health (e.g. anorexia nervosa)
Low	Low	Normal	Decreased TBP*
Low	Low	High	Hypothyroidism

*TBP = thyroxine binding protein

Table 2 summarizes some of the results that may be obtained by measuring the total T_4, total T_3 and TSH levels. The significance of the various combinations is indicated in this table and more detailed accounts of these results are given in later chapters. Causes for increased thyroxine-binding protein levels, which will increase the total T_4 level, have already been shown in Table 1, as well as drugs which may occupy the thyroxine-binding sites on the carrier proteins and give rise to lowered total serum T_4 levels. A low or absent thyroxine-binding globulin level may occur as an

innocent congenital abnormality. This abnormality is related
to the X chromosome which determines whether a fetus is
male or female. Because of this, deficient thyroxine-binding
globulin and hence a low total T_4 level is usually found only
in males. Although such men have low T_4 and T_3 levels,
because the carrier-protein is reduced, they have a normal
amount of free thyroxine (and T_3) and are euthyroid.

Thyrotrophin-releasing hormone (*TRH*) *test.* This test is only
used in instances when there is doubt as to whether or not
the thyroid gland is overactive or underactive. It is particularly
helpful in confirming the diagnosis of hyperthyroidism or
hypothyroidism when the T_4 level is at or just above or just
below the normal range. This test is also of some value in
determining the cause of certain changes in the eyes which,
although often associated with hyperthyroidism in patients
with Graves' disease, may occasionally occur before there is
any clinical evidence of thyroid overactivity (p. 38). This
TRH test is also used to distinguish primary failure of the
thyroid from that which much less often occurs secondarily
to disease of either the pituitary or hypothalamic gland whereby the secretion of TSH is reduced to negligible amounts.
   The main inconvenience of the test is that it takes about
$1\frac{1}{2}$ hours to perform. First a sample of blood is taken to
determine the TSH level. Thyrotrophin-releasing hormone is
then injected intravenously. Minor and very temporary side-
effects may be experienced by the patient. In about 50 per
cent of cases, the patient experiences for a few seconds
mild nausea, a metallic taste in the mouth, flushing of the
face, and a sensation between the legs which for a moment
may bring an urge to pass urine.
   Further blood samples for TSH are taken 20 and 60
minutes after the TRH injection. As shown in Fig. 4 the
resultant responses in the TSH levels allows a clear distinction
between the hypothyroid patient with primary thyroid gland
failure and the normal euthyroid subject. In the hypothyroid

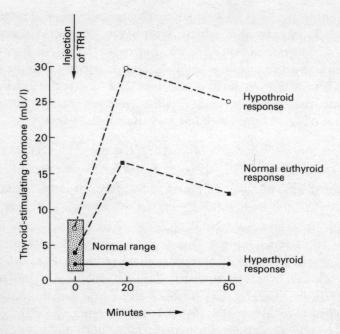

Fig. 4. The response of the level of thyroid stimulating hormone (TSH) to the intravenous injection of thyrotrophin-releasing hormone (TRH) in hypothyroid, hyperthyroid, and normal subjects.

patient (Chapter 7) the thyrotrophin (TSH)-forming cells in the pituitary are enlarged in size and secretory activity in an attempt to keep the failing thyroid gland working. Because of this the pituitary cells secreting TSH respond to the releasing hormone (TRH) by secreting a greater than normal amount of TSH (Fig. 4). Thus at 20 minutes there is an exaggerated rise in the TSH level which increases to 20 milliunits/litre or higher but drops back a little at 60 minutes. In patients with hypothalamic or pituitary disease causing secondary failure of thyroid secretion there is often a delayed TSH response to TRH whereby the TSH level at 60 minutes is greater than that at 20 minutes.

Conversely in hyperthyroidism (Chapter 4) the pituitary's secretion of thyrotrophin (TSH) is abnormally suppressed.

24

Investigation of thyroid disorders

The pituitary is so inactive in its output of TSH that when thyrotrophin-releasing hormone (TRH) is injected, the TSH level in the patient's serum remains unaffected (Fig. 4) and at 20 and 60 minutes does not increase above the low initial (basal) level by more than about 1 milliunit/litre — an absent or impaired response. A similar result is obtained in about 50–75 per cent of patients with the eye complications of Graves' disease even though there is no hyperthyroidism judging by the normal levels of T_4 and T_3 (p. 40).

Tests to determine the cause of thyroid disease

These investigations are directed at finding out why the thyroid is abnormal. They help to decide why the gland is, for example, underactive. This may be obvious if the patient has had a surgical subtotal thyroidectomy — too much of the gland has been removed — or if the patient with previous hyperthyroidism has been treated with radioactive iodine. In less obvious cases the cause may lie in maldevelopment of the gland in childhood, in destruction of the gland associated with thyroid antibodies (Hashimoto's thyroiditis), in iodine deficiency, or to abnormality or deficiency of one of the biochemical steps needed to manufacture T_4 or T_3 in the thyroid cells.

Such investigations may help to decide if a lump in the gland is a hollow cyst or a solid nodule, and whether it is benign (non-cancerous) or malignant.

Investigations may be necessary to determine whether hyperthyroidism is due to an autoimmune process that induces the whole gland to produce excess thyroid hormones or whether it is due to a localized area of overactive cells secreting too much hormone (toxic adenoma). All these distinctions are important because they may have a significant bearing on how the patient is best treated.

Radio-isotope thyroid scan. In this investigation the patient is given a radio-isotope that is selectively taken up by the thyroid gland. The gland becomes temporarily radioactive, and this radioactivity is charted by a counter placed over the neck in the region of the gland. Various isotopes of iodine may be given for this test but most often a man-made element, technetium, is used. The amount of radioactive material given is a very small tracer quantity, and the patient need have no fears as to the radiation dose, which is minute. The external counter placed over the neck maps out the thyroid gland and the resulting picture may be in black and white on an X-ray film or in colour as shown in Plate 1 (reproduced in black and white).

A normal thyroid isotope scan will show the right and left lobes; not always does it show the isthmus. The gland is located in the correct position in the neck and the two lobes are of approximately equal size. The uptake of isotope is uniform throughout the lobes but radioactivity is greater in the centre of each lobe than at the periphery because there is more thyroid tissue in the middle of the lobe.

Maldevelopment. If the thyroid gland does not develop properly in fetal life and does not descend as it should from its origin at the base of the tongue downwards into the neck, a thyroid isotope scan will show this. What little radioactivity there is will be located high in the neck under the chin. This is mainly of importance when seeking the cause of thyroid deficiency in a baby or young child.

Sometimes the thyroid descends too far. The scan will usually show some activity in the lower part of the neck but the greater part of the gland lies behind the breastbone in the upper part of the chest (a retrosternal goitre).

In the hyperthyroidism the isotope scan may show one of three appearances. (1) In Graves' disease the whole gland is overactive: thus the scan shows high isotope activity uniformly throughout both lobes, and usually the lobes are increased in size. (2) When hyperthyroidism is caused by overactivity of a small clump (a toxic adenoma) of cells, the radioactivity is largely or totally confined to this hyperactive area (Plate 2). This is often called a 'hot' nodule because of the excess uptake of iostope in one area. The rest of the thyroid takes up little or no isotope and is 'cold' because it is inactive. This results from excess T_4 and T_3 being formed by the 'hot' toxic nodule, and hence the secretion of TSH from the pituitary is switched off by the normal feedback mechanism. Because no TSH is being secreted, the thyroid gland, except for the 'hot' nodule, becomes inactive and does not take up the isotope. (3) In a multinodular toxic goitre the activity of the gland is confined to a number of different areas in the thyroid which may vary in size and degree of activity. This is reflected in the scan which shows multiple 'hot' nodules separated by areas of inactive ('cold') tissue.

The distinction between hyperthyroidism due to Graves' disease and that caused by a solitary 'hot' nodule can often be made on clinical grounds but if there is doubt an isotope scan will make the differentiation which is important from the point of view of choosing the correct treatment (see Chapter 4).

An isotope scan is also useful in determining the nature of a lump in the thyroid gland. Quite often one sees a patient who has noticed a painless lump — perhaps the size of a grape — in her neck. On examination this lump is found to be part of the thyroid gland; it moves on swallowing with the rest of the gland, which otherwise feels perfectly normal. An isotope scan may show that this nodule takes up the radioactive tracer, in which case it is virtually certain that the nodule is not cancerous. On the other hand the scan may show that the nodule does not take up the isotope. In other words it is a 'cold' nodule (Plate 3). This makes it more likely that the nodule is malignant, but in fact most — about 75 per cent — 'cold' nodules when removed and examined under the microscope fortunately prove not to be malignant. Sometimes an isotope scan done to investigate what appears on examination to be a solitary nodule shows that not only is the nodule 'cold' but that there are other 'cold' areas in the rest of the thyroid which felt normal. This is a helpful finding because it shows that the patient has multiple 'cold' nodules, not a solitary nodule, and this makes it much less likely that malignant change has occurred.

Isotope scanning, with radio-iodine rather than technetium, is invaluable in the management of patients with thyroid cancer (Chapter 9).

Ultrasound scan. Concern over the nature of a solitary nodule — as to whether it is benign or malignant — has led to the use of other techniques that may prove helpful. One such is the ultrasound scan, which is totally painless. A probe is placed over the thyroid gland and an inaudible 'sound' wave sent through the skin and into the thyroid tissue. This wave is reflected back to a receiver in the probe and recorded. As the probe is moved from side to side over the gland a pattern emerges (Plate 4), just as when this technique is used for locating a submarine or wreck on the seabed. The ultrasound scan will show whether the nodule is composed of solid tissue or whether it is hollow and filled with fluid, i.e. it is a cyst in the thyroid. Cysts are seldom malignant.

Needle-biopsy. Although painless non-invasive procedures such as an isotope and an ultrasound scan are preferred for investigating the nature of a thyroid lump, sometimes they fail to provide the necessary data to decide whether the nodule is benign or malignant. Nor can these non-invasive techniques always be relied upon because absolute certainty as to the nature of a lump can only be established by examining the cells under a microscope. Although a safe decision may be made on the evidence of isotope and ultrasound scans, if any doubt persists some tissue must be obtained for microscopical examination. This can be attempted by a needle or drill biopsy. The overlying skin and the fatty tissue underneath it are usually injected with local anaesthetic, in much the same way as a dentist anaesthetizes a tooth. A needle or a little circular drill is then passed through the anaesthetized area into the nodule and a core of tissue is removed. This procedure is not painful, although some patients understandably find it rather frightening to have a needle pushed into their neck. The disadvantages of a needle biopsy are that the core of tissue obtained may be too small for the pathologist who examines it under the microscope to express a firm opinion as to whether the cells are benign or malignant, and the tissue removed may not be representative of the whole nodule.

Open or surgical biopsy. In most instances when there is continuing doubt as to the nature of a nodule, an open biopsy under a general anaesthetic is done by a surgeon. This provides both a firm pathological diagnosis and a cure because the whole of the lump in question is removed.

Thyroid auto-antibodies. As explained on page 9 in Chapter 2, antibodies may develop in the body which act on the cells of the thyroid gland. These antibodies may be of several different types and react with different components of the thyroid gland. Those antibodies associated with destruction of thyroid cells, such as occurs in Hashimoto's thyroiditis, can readily be detected in the bloodstream and their strength can be measured. The most common are those directed against thyroglobulin and microsomes, which are a constituent of thyroid cells. Various techniques of increasing sensitivity (precipitin, latex, compliment fixation, tanned red cells, immunofluorescence, and competitive binding radioassay tests) are used for detecting and quantifying these.

It is not enough to decide that a patient has hypothyroidism by doing studies of thyroid secretory function and finding that the T_4 is low and the TSH level is high. The next question should be 'why is this patient thyroid deficient?', and the most common cause is autoimmune destruction of the thyroid associated with antibodies which are found in high titre in the serum. Autoimmune destruction of the thyroid gland is a slow process that may take place over many months or years. Sometimes the antibodies are found long before there is thyroid failure. At the present time we do not have a safe and effective way of arresting the destructive process but the knowledge that these antibodies are present will ensure that a careful eye is kept on the patient so that corrective thyroxine replacement therapy is given as soon as, or even before, the thyroid ceases to secrete an adequate normal amount of thyroxine.

It is important to know the cause of hypothyroidism because autoimmune destruction of the thyroid gland is quite often associated with other autoimmune diseases. For example about 10 per cent of patients with Hashimoto's hypothyroidism develop pernicious anaemia. Because this is easily treatable it is no longer properly called 'pernicious' anaemia. It is the result of vitamin B_{12} deficiency. Vitamin B_{12} is absorbed from the intestine by interaction with a substance (intrinsic factor) secreted by certain cells (the parietal cells) in the stomach wall. In patients who have, or may later develop, pernicious anaemia, auto-antibodies to the gastric parietal cells are often found in the blood. Thus in patients with autoimmune hypothyroidism, a search for gastric parietal antibodies should be made. If present, the patient's haemoglobin must be watched and the development of pernicious anaemia treated by injections of vitamin B_{12} every six weeks.

Techniques for detecting the thyroid-stimulating antibodies that cause Graves' disease (primary hyperthyroidism) are at present only done in a few research laboratories. It is hoped that the procedure will become more widely available. By the present procedures thyroid-stimulating antibodies are found in 80 per cent of patients with Graves' disease and in 60 per cent of euthyroid patients with eye complications of the condition (Graves' ophthalmopathy, see p. 38).

Investigation of thyroid disorders

X-rays. Conventional X-ray pictures are of limited use in the investigation of thyroid diseases. When there is a large goitre the degree of compression or deviation of the windpipe can be determined by radiographs of the neck. A retrosternal goitre may be suspected from a shadow seen in the upper part of a chest X-ray, and confirmed by an isotope scan.

Computer-assisted tomography (CAT or CT scan) of the eyes and the bony sockets in which they lie is helpful to determine the nature of eye changes suggestive of Graves' ophthalmopathy especially when these changes are confined to one eye only (p. 40).

4

Hyperthyroidism

Hyperthyroidism, also known as thyrotoxicosis, is a clinical state in which increased amounts of the two thyroid hormones — thyroxine (T_4) and triiodothyronine (T_3) — are usually present in the bloodstream. Sometimes only the T_3 level is raised — so-called T_3 toxicosis.

Causes of hyperthyroidism

The causes of hyperthyroidism are many (Table 3) but in practice 99 per cent of cases are caused by increased secretion of hormones from a gland that is being overstimulated by thyroid-stimulating antibodies (Graves' disease or diffuse toxic goitre) or that is the site of one or more toxic nodules.

The commonest cause of hyperthyroidism is Graves' disease. Because all the thyroid cells are made overactive by stimulating antibodies circulating in the bloodstream, the whole gland is hyperactive, and this is shown by a radioactive isotope scan in which the isotope is found uniformly distributed throughout both lobes. The gland is usually symmetrically enlarged to a moderate degree although it may

Table 3 *Causes of hyperthyroidism*

Graves' disease (diffuse toxic goitre)

Toxic nodular goitre — multinodular (Plummer's disease) or uninodular (toxic adenoma)

Excessive dosage with T_4 or T_3

Iodide medication (Jod–Basedow phenomenon)

Thyroiditis (viral or Hashimoto's) causing transient thyrotoxicosis

Excess TSH or related hormone secretion

range from being normal in size to visually obvious enlargement. Certain changes often occur in the eyes of a patient with this primary hyperthyroidism (Graves' disease) and these will be described later.

The second most common cause of hyperthyroidism is a toxic nodular goitre, and the gland may contain several nodules (multinodular toxic goitre, also known as Plummer's disease) or only one (toxic adenoma). A toxic adenoma is a clump of cells which can often be felt as a nodule 1–2 cm in diameter. Such a nodule is not malignant and is called toxic because it elaborates excess thyroid hormones and thus induces thyrotoxicosis. Toxic adenomas tend to develop in thyroid glands that have previously, often for many years, been enlarged and already contain other nodules. Thus this type of thyrotoxicosis is often called secondary hyperthyroidism, because the overactivity is secondary to a previous thyroid disorder. Hyperthyroidism due to toxic nodules tends to occur in patients who are in late middle-age or older, and it is not accompanied by the important eye changes that may occur in patients with primary hyperthyroidism (Graves' disease).

Hyperthyroidism may occur if a patient is given too much thyroxine or triiodothyronine for the correction of thyroid deficiency (Chapter 7). Hypothyroid patients who become depressed often take an excessive amount of T_4 in a vain attempt to increase their flagging energy. Some obese people think that, because patients with hyperthyroidism usually lose weight, they too will become thinner if they take thyroxine. If a person with a normal thyroid gland takes thyroxine in small or moderate dosage, this extra thyroxine will switch off the secretion of thyrotrophin-releasing hormone from the hypothalamus and of thyroid-stimulating hormone from the pituitary (Fig. 2). Their own thyroid gland will no longer be stimulated, and its secretion of T_4 and T_3 will drop off. With the gland in a resting state, the levels of T_4 and T_3 in the bloodstream will be maintained within the normal range largely by the contribution from the thyroxine which the patient is taking in tablet form by mouth. Thus to induce abnormally high blood levels of T_4 and T_3 a normal person has to take excessive amounts of thyroxine or triiodothyronine by mouth, with the attendant risks that accompany hyperthyroidism.

Very rarely certain iodine-containing medicines, particularly if taken for a long time, induce hyperthyroidism in predisposed subjects. This is known as the Jod–Basedow phenomenon. Most often it occurs in patients who live in an iodine-deficient part of the world and already have a goitre. Presumably they have occult Graves' disease or a toxic nodular goitre but cannot become hyperthyroid until they are given iodine and can then manufacture excess T_4 or T_3 or both.

Transient hyperthyroidism may occur during the course of thyroiditis whether this is caused by a virus (Chapter 5) or by Hashimoto's autoimmune disease (Chapter 6).

Very rarely indeed is hyperthyroidism caused by excessive secretion of TSH from a pituitary tumour. Slightly less rare but very uncommon is the development of thyroid gland overactivity in a woman with a hydatidiform mole in the uterus or in a man with a cancer (choriocarcinoma) of the testis. Both these tumours may secrete an excess of a hormone (chorionic gonadotrophin) which acts on the thyroid gland like TSH does.

Graves' disease

Thyrotoxicosis due to Graves' disease occurs ten times more commonly in women than in men but the reason for this is not known. It tends to run in families and those with a particular constitutional body cell type (HLA B8-DRW3) seem most vulnerable. What triggers off the disease is unknown. In some instances Graves' disease seems to follow an emotional upset but it has not proved possible to establish scientific proof of such a cause-and-effect relationship. For instance during the present troubles in Northern Ireland which started in 1968 there has been no significant increase in the incidence of Graves' disease there.

The condition usually comes on slowly, and it may be several months before the patient realizes she is ill.

Graves' disease usually occurs in women aged 18–40. Younger girls of 5 or more may develop the condition. It may occur in older patients of either sex and very rarely as neonatal thyrotoxicosis in a baby born to a mother who has, or has had in the past, Graves' disease.

Tiredness is usually the first symptom, to be followed by weight loss, palpitations of the heart or consciousness of the heart's action, nervousness, apprehension or irritability, and increased sweating. The patient feels hot all the time and is uncomfortable in warm weather. There is often generalized itching of the skin (pruritus). The tiredness may become profound and the patient notices shortness of breath on hurrying or climbing a flight of stairs. There is a tendency to looseness of the bowels and sometimes to frank diarrhoea. When asked the patient may say her appetite has increased and the house-keeping cost has risen in consequence; but despite a voracious appetite most patients quickly lose 7lb (3 kg) to 21 lb (9.5 kg) in weight. Menstruation tends to become less heavy and periods may be missed or even stop.

The eye complications, perhaps better called the associated eye problems, are often the first and most obvious manifestation of Graves' disease. The eyes appear starey because the upper lid is pulled upwards and the white of the eyes is more prominent just as when an actress wishes to convey fear or terror. The eyes may also bulge outwards. These and other aspects of the eye problems that are peculiar to Graves' disease are discussed below.

Hyperthyroidism in patients aged 55 or more may present in a rather different way from that in the younger patient. The very typical features described above are less apparent and the brunt of the disease falls upon the heart. This is particularly so in the patient with a toxic adenoma who tends to be in the older age group.

Multinodular and uninodular toxic goitre

In these conditions the clinical picture is much the same as in Graves' disease except that the patient is usually older and the goitre may be quite large. The gland feels nodular and an isotope scan will show increased uptake in one or more of the nodules. Sometimes the activity is most marked in the tissue between the nodules and this finding suggests that Graves' disease has developed in a previously multinodular gland.

Often the heart is affected at an early stage. Neglected or inadequately treated Graves' disease will eventually affect the heart too but because patients with a toxic nodule or nodules tend to be older they usually present with shortness of breath, tiredness, and swelling of the ankles — all symptoms, when taken in combination, of heart failure. The patient may notice an irregular pounding of the heart due to the onset of atrial fibrillation: in this the electrical control of the heartbeat is disturbed and the heart does not contract in an even rhythmical manner. The other features of hyperthyroidism may be present in greater or lesser degree. Weight loss usually occurs but this tends to be less striking than in Graves' disease because the retention of fluid, responsible for the ankle swelling and the shortness of breath, offsets to some extent the reduction of weight caused by increased metabolism with the loss of fat and muscle.

What the doctor finds

Patients with hyperthyroidism are usually thin or show evidence of weight loss. They are restless and anxious. It is hard for them to sit still and they fidget in the chair plucking at their handbag or twiddling their fingers. Children tend to be clumsy and drop things. Even on a cold day they are lightly

36

clad. Their hands are hot and when held outstretched there is a fine tremor — not a coarse shaking. The pulse rate is fast: this may be due to 'natural' nervousness but in fact the fast rate is persistent and in the old days when thyrotoxic patients were admitted to hospital the sleeping pulse rate, taken by the night nurses, was also fast.

The thyroid gland may be of normal size but usually it is slightly enlarged and may be quite big in a multinodular toxic goitre. Because it is overactive and producing too much thyroid hormone, the blood flow through the gland is increased. This is detected as a swishing murmur when a stethoscope is held over the front of the neck. The doctor will ask you to stop breathing when he does this, otherwise he will be deafened by the noise of air going up and down the windpipe.

Often the patient has starey eyes and this may be the first sign that alerts the doctor to the diagnosis.

Muscular weakness may not have been noticed by the patient but can be obvious to the doctor. The most affected are the muscles of shoulder and pelvic girdles and this is more common in men than women. Thus the patient may not be able to raise his arms against slight resistance or he may have difficulty in getting up from a lying position on the floor. An even more severe type of periodic paralysis may occur particularly in Chinese or Japanese patients with thyrotoxicosis.

Some patients, particularly those with the eye complications (see below), develop curious areas of thickened skin on the lower part of the legs. This is called *pretibial myxoedema*. It may occur early in Graves' disease but more often comes on about one year after the condition has been treated and is more common after radioiodine than surgical treatment. First an area of the skin becomes reddened, and then the skin becomes thickened. Hair growing in the affected area becomes coarse. The area of affected skin tends to increase in size; new areas may develop and sometimes the top of the foot or of the big toe becomes involved.

Associated changes in the eyes. Minor degrees of involvement of the eyes are common in hyperthyroidism. There is a tendency for the upper eyelids to be pulled upwards (Plate 5), and when the patient looks down the upper lids are slow to follow the eyeballs (Plate 6). Thus the eyes develop a staring quality. This appearance is due to changes in the nervous control of the upper eyelid and usually disappears as the hyperthyroidism is controlled. These changes may occur in hyperthyroidism due to any cause, and are not specific to Graves' disease.

More troublesome eye changes may occur in Graves' disease and virtually never develop in any other type of thyroid disease. The relationship between Graves' disease and these more severe eye changes is complex. Some patients with Graves' disease never develop eye complications and there is no correlation between the severity of the thyrotoxicosis and the liability to eye changes. Others develop them without ever becoming hyperthyroid — so-called Graves' or dysthyroid ophthalmopathy. In others the eye complications precede the hyperthyroidism, start concurrently with the symptoms and signs (and laboratory confirmation) of thyrotoxicosis, or occur only after the hyperthyroidism has been successfully treated and the patient rendered euthyroid. Furthermore the eye changes may be confined to one eye or occur first in one eye and then in the other. When both eyes are involved, one may be worse than the other.

There has been much dispute as to the cause of the eye complications. It is agreed that the fundamental abnormality is an increase in the bulk of tissue in the bony sockets in which the eyes lie. What is contentious is the mechanism for this increase in intra-orbital tissue which causes protrusion of the eyes (proptosis or exophthalmos), impedes the drainage of fluid from the eyelids, and by increasing the pressure in the rigid eye-sockets may impair the conducting function of the optic nerves which carry light appreciation or vision from the eyes to the brain.

The most widely accepted explanation is that lymphocyte white cells and antibodies similar to, but not identical with, those that stimulate the thyroid cells in Graves' disease attack the muscles that move the eyes and increase the bulk of tissue that occupies the sockets in which the eyeballs are housed.

As a consequence drainage of fluid is impaired and there is deposition of fatty material in the upper or lower eyelids, or both (Class 2 changes in Table 4). The upper lid bulges forwards

Table 4 *Eye changes associated with thyroid disease* (classification of the American Thyroid Association)

Class 1	Lid retraction and lid lag
Class 2	Soft tissue swelling of upper and/or lower lids Swelling of the conjunctiva (chemosis) Prominence of the outer scleral veins
Class 3	Protrusion of the eyeball (proptosis or exophthalmos)
Class 4	Paralysis of muscles that move the eyes (oculomotor palsy; ophthalmoplegia)
Class 5	Inflammation of the cornea
Class 6	Involvement of the optic nerve (optic atrophy; papilloedema)

Class 2–6 changes are specific to Graves' disease or to Graves' ophthalmopathy.

and 'bags' develop under the eyes, which may be so large that they hang like sacks over the cheeks. Drainage from the front of the eye is impeded; the membraneous covering of the eye (the conjunctiva) becomes waterlogged and the resulting 'chemosis' makes the eyes look watery. The veins that drain blood from the front of the eye become engorged and show up prominently on the outer side of each eyeball (scleral injection).

The increase of tissue within the orbital cavities pushes the eyes forwards, a condition known as proptosis or exophthalmos (Plate 7). In more severe cases the muscles that

move the eyeball are so involved that the patient is unable
to look upwards without tilting the head back and later
may have restriction of eye movement from side to side
(oculomotor palsy or ophthalmoplegia). This often results in
double vision (diplopia). When looking straight ahead the
patient will see one finger; when she looks upwards or to
one side she will see two fingers. This type of infiltrative
ophthalmpathy — so-called because the orbit is invaded by
inflammatory cells — may affect one or both eyes or one
eye more than the other. Because the eyeball is pushed
forward, it is less protected by the lids and is more liable
to be irritated by dust or wind. Thus the eye tends to water
excessively and the patient experiences a feeling of grittiness
in the eye due to inflammation of the cornea — another
outer covering of the eye (Table 4). In very severe cases
the cornea is liable to infection which may impair vision.
Sometimes, though rarely, the raised pressure in the bony
orbit may damage the optic nerve that conveys the visual
image to the brain. Such changes — infection of the exposed
front of the eye, marked exophthalmos, and actual or potential
damage to the optic nerve — constitute 'malignant exophthalmos' (Plate 8), not a good term because the condition has
nothing to do with cancer although it is serious ('malignant')
in that the patient, if untreated, may go blind. These more
severe eye complications are often more troublesome in men
than in women.

When the eye features occur months or years before
hyperthyroidism (and in some cases hyperthyroidism never
develops) it may be difficult to decide whether they are those
associated with Graves' disease, because features of overactivity of the thyroid gland have not emerged, or whether
they are due to some local abnormality in the orbit. The
problem is all the more difficult when only one eye is involved
(unilateral as opposed to bilateral exophthalmos). The finding
of thyroid auto-antibodies in the patient's blood makes
Graves' ophthalmopathy likely even though the T_4 or T_3

levels, or both, are normal: in fact about 60–70 per cent of euthyroid patients with ophthalmopathy have thyroglobulin or microsomal antibodies, or both. About half the patients who have the ophthalmic manifestations of Graves' disease before they develop evidence of hyperthyroidism have an abnormal TRH test (Fig. 4): the TSH level remains flat when TRH is injected intravenously (p. 25). Special X-rays of the orbit and the eyeball can be helpful. These computerized or computer-assisted pictures taken at sliced intervals (p. 31) show what is going on in the orbit. In the ophthalmic form of Graves' disease the tissues in the orbit are increased in bulk and there is a characteristic thickening of some or all of the muscles that regulate the movement of the eyeballs (Plate 9).

There is much we do not understand about the factors that produce these eye complications. Although treatment will save sight and mitigate the symptoms, the cosmetic result — the appearance of the eyes — may fall short of what the patient would like. There is a belief among some doctors that antithyroid treatment which suddenly reduces the bloodstream level of thyroxine may aggravate or worsen the eye features. This belief has not been proved conclusively, but it implies that when eye symptoms are prominent it is prudent to treat the associated hyperthyroidism gently. It is certainly important not to overtreat the hyperthyroid patient so that they become hypothyroid when there seems increased likelihood of the eye features becoming worse. With proper supervision, and replacement treatment with thyroxine when there is any risk of hypothyroidism developing, this should not occur.

Diagnosis of hyperthyroidism

In its early stages the diagnosis of thyroid gland overactivity can be difficult. The problem is less evident later in the course of the disease when the clinical picture is more florid. Hyperthyroidism has to be distinguished from anxiety, the cause of which may be known to, and recognized by, the patient or may be unknown and therefore unconscious to her. This distinction from anxiety can be difficult in making a diagnosis because hyperthyroidism certainly in the younger patient is often accompanied by anxiety. It is not simply a matter of distinguishing between hyperthyroidism and anxiety; it is a matter of distinguishing between (anxiety) and (hyperthyroidism + anxiety). These conditions have much in common but laboratory tests will make the distinction and in anxiety the physical accompaniments such as weight loss, a fine tremor (not coarse shakiness) of the hands, and clinical evidence of increased metabolism are usually less prominent.

In the older patient hyperthyroidism may have to be distinguished from depression with associated agitation. This can be difficult for the doctor because many of the same symptoms are common to hyperthyroidism and agitated depression. Again laboratory tests will make the distinction.

In the even older patient who presents with constant irregularity of the pulse (atrial fibrillation), shortness of breath, pain in the centre of the chest on exertion (angina), and ankle swelling the possibility of hyperthyroidism, usually due to a multinodular goitre or a toxic adenoma, may need to be considered. Erroneously sometimes the atrial fibrillation and the heart failure are attributed to high blood pressure or to narrowing of the coronary arteries that carry blood to the muscle of the heart. Unless it can be certain that the high blood pressure or the coronary artery disease is predominant, the doctor will wish to make sure that the patient is not hyperthyroid.

Hyperthyroidism is more common in women. There is often a family history – in parents, brothers or sisters, grandparents, aunts and uncles – of some thyroid disease be it an enlargement of the thyroid gland (goitre), hyperthyroidism, or hypothyroidism.

Fortunately laboratory tests usually give clear-cut results

in deciding whether a patient is hyperthyroid or not. In most instances the serum thyroxine level is unequivocally raised above normal. In rare patients — often only in the early phases — the T_4 is normal but the T_3 level is raised (T_3 toxicosis). Difficulties in interpreting the T_4 level may arise when the carrier-protein is increased as in women taking oestrogens in any form (such as the oral contraceptive) or when they are pregnant (p. 17). In these cases or when certain drugs are being taken (p. 18) more complex tests may be necessary to measure directly or indirectly the amount of carrier-protein present (for example the T_3 resin-binding test) so that the true level of free unbound-to-protein thyroxine can be calculated by the 'free thyroxine index' (see p. 20).

In extreme cases of doubt the TRH test (p. 23) will prove helpful as may a thyroid isotope scan. However in the early stages of hyperthyroidism nothing is lost by keeping the patient under observation and using time as a diagnostic ally. The clinical picture, and hence the diagnosis, is likely to become clearer over a few weeks or months of careful observation, and after this time the laboratory tests will become unequivocally abnormal.

Treatment

Left untreated patients with Graves' disease run a fluctuating course with temporary — rarely permanent — remissions and relapses. In patients with a multinodular goitre or a toxic adenoma remissions are uncommon. The overall mortality of untreated thyrotoxicosis in the old days was about 25 per cent. Thus the condition must always be treated.

There are three main methods of treating hyperthyroidism. These are (1) antithyroid drugs which suppress the ability of the thyroid gland to make T_4 and T_3, (2) surgical removal of most of the thyroid gland (subtotal thyroidectomy), and (3) radio-iodine (^{131}I) which is concentrated in the cells of the thyroid gland and by irradiation destroys them. Which of these three methods is used depends upon a considerable number of factors which have to be considered in each individual case. The more important of these factors can be listed:

(1) whether the hyperthyroidism is due to Graves' disease, a multinodular goitre or a toxic adenoma;
(2) the age of the patient;
(3) the sex of the patient;
(4) whether the thyroid gland is large or not, and whether it is cosmetically unsightly;
(5) whether the thyroid gland is located in the neck in the normal place or is retrosternal;
(6) the patient's wishes, personality, and occupation;
(7) whether it is possible for the patient to remain under intermittent but prolonged medical supervision or whether they want a rapid and once-and-for-all cure;
(8) whether an experienced thyroid surgeon is available;
(9) what previous method of treatment has been used.

The relevance of these factors will become apparent later.

Two other treatments, that relieve the patient's hyperthyroid symptoms but which do not permanently cure the condition, are important.

Beta-blocking drugs, such as propranolol, reduce the tremor of the patient's hands, the sweating, the agitation or nervousness, and the palpitations and fast heart-rate. Propranolol is a very safe drug and is most useful in making the patient feel more comfortable until control of the hyperthyroidism or a definitive cure has been achieved. The correct dose is that which satisfactorily slows the rapid heartbeat and makes the patient generally feel more comfortable. The important thing that the patient must know is that it may be dangerous to stop taking these tablets suddenly. Thus the patient must not run out of the tablets, and when there is no longer need for a beta-blocker, the dosage should gradually be reduced and then stopped.

Iodine has a temporary suppressive effect on the thyroid gland. This effect lasts for only about three weeks. In the present-day management of hyperthyroidism, iodine, usually in the form of drops of Lugol's iodine taken in a little milk three times daily, is reserved for the preparation of the patient before subtotal surgical removal of the gland. The usual practice is to start the Lugol's iodine 7–14 days before the time of the operation.

Antithyroid drugs

A number of related compounds suppress the manufacture of T_4 and T_3 by the thyroid cells. Treatment with these drugs reduces the synthesis of thyroid hormones and renders the patient euthyorid. If the drug is given in too large a dose for too long a time the patient will actually become hypothyroid. Thus the dosage must be adjusted to the patient's response as judged clinically by the doctor and also by the thyroid hormone level in the bloodstream. Often it is simpler to give a fairly large continuous dose of the antithyroid drug and prevent the patient from becoming hypothyroid by adding later a small amount of thyroxine.

Antithyroid drugs will certainly render the patient euthyroid but they may not cure the underlying disease because when the drug is stopped, the hyperthyroidism may gradually over the next 3–12 months recur. This is almost invariably the case in a patient with a multinodular toxic goitre or a toxic adenoma, and hence except as a temporary measure hyperthyroidism due to these two causes is best treated by surgery or radio-iodine.

In Graves' disease treatment with antithyroid drugs for 18–24 months induces a permanent remission in about 50 per cent of patients. We are not sure why some patients respond so favourably whereas the other 50 per cent in a matter of months after stopping treatment get a return of their hyperthyroidism. Patients with a mild degree of thyroid overactivity, with a normal sized or only slightly enlarged gland and those who are treated at an early stage are usually found in the group that have a permanent remission in response to antithyroid drug treatment. Conversely those who have large glands, are severely thyrotoxic, and in whom there has been some delay in initiating treatment are more liable to relapse when the antithyroid treatment is stopped. But the size of the goitre and the severity of the hyperthyroidism are certainly not the only factors that determine the long-term response to antithyroid drugs. In addition to suppressing the synthesis of T_4 and T_3 in the thyroid cells, antithyroid drugs also seem to have an effect on the basic causation of Graves' disease. They decrease the level in the bloodstream of the thyroid-stimulating antibodies and it is the level of these antibodies after 18 months of antithyroid treatment that appears to determine whether or not the patient will stay in remission and remain euthyroid, or whether the patient will relapse and become hyperthyroid again.

A relapse after antithyroid medical treatment is not a disaster. It simply prolongs the period of medical supervision until the patient is rendered euthyroid by subtotal thyroid-ectomy or radio-iodine. Which of these two is used, largely decided according to the patient's age and sex, is discussed later. These methods are used because experience has shown that failure of one course of medical treatment, i.e. a relapse after stopping antithyroid drugs, is nearly always followed by further relapses after second or third courses of antithyroid drugs.

Antithyroid drugs are used for the treatment of those rare cases of hyperthyroidism occurring in new-born babies (Chapter 10). It is also the best treatment for children with Graves' disease. Children with thyrotoxicosis very seldom experience a permanent remission after antithyroid drugs. They nearly always relapse when the treatment is stopped.

Thus the usual practice is to continue antithyroid drugs (with or without additional thyroxine to keep the child euthyroid) until the patient reaches the age of 18–20 years. Then when they are grown up, have finished school, and before going to university or starting their first job, a subtotal thyroidectomy is done.

Antithyroid drugs are used in patients with Graves' disease of either sex aged 20–40, particularly if the gland is not large and the degree of hyperthyroidism not great. Because of the approximately 50 per cent failure rate this may not always be the optimal treatment for women who are married, contemplate marriage, or wish to start a family. Hypethyroidism often reduces the frequency of menstruation, and temporary infertility is common in thyrotoxic women. With medical treatment with antithyroid drugs the patient becomes euthyroid. She then marries and wishes to start a family. She may become hyperthyroid again while she is pregnant. This does not present insurmountable problems although there is a somewhat increased risk of miscarriage. During pregnancy antithyroid drugs in small dosage can be given without damage to the fetus in the womb, provided that the treatment is stopped 4–6 weeks before the baby is born. Having had the baby, the mother needs to re-start antithyroid medication but this may be secreted in her milk and conventionally prevents her from breast-feeding. Life is not made easier when the patient, in addition to looking after her newly arrived baby, has to go to the doctor to have the treatment of her Graves' disease supervised. These difficulties can largely be avoided if surgical treatment is used in young women facing the prospect of marriage and having children.

As mentioned earlier a relatively rapid reduction in the thyroid hormone level seems to aggravate the eye complications in some patients with Graves' disease. For this reason initial treatment with antithyroid drugs is often used to assess the effect of this on the eye changes, before it is decided whether to go ahead with definitive curative treatment with either surgery or radio-iodine.

Long-term antithyroid drug treatment for 18–24 months should not be used in patients whose occupation prevents them from remaining under regular medical supervision, nor should it be used for those who cannot be relied upon to take their tablets regularly. Surgery is best for those who must have a rapid once-and-for-all cure, for those with an unsightly large gland, for those with a retrosternal toxic goitre, and when the thyroid is causing serious displacement or compression of the windpipe of sufficient degree to interfere with breathing.

Antithyroid preparations and side effects

The three most commonly used antithyroid drugs are carbimazole, methimazole, and propylthiouracil (see Glossary, p. 108). There is not much to chose between them but carbimazole and methimazole are the most widely used, the latter particularly in North America. Side effects are very uncommon, and when they do occur it is usually during the first two months of treatment. In order of frequency the side effects of carbimazole and methimazole are nausea or mild indigestion and skin rashes, followed by an unusual combination of pain in the joints, a low temperature, and sometimes swelling of the lymphatic glands. These reactions disappear quickly when the drug is stopped and may not recur if propylthiouracil is given.

The most serious side effect of any of these preparations is agranulocytosis. For reasons that are not known – and fortunately it is extremely rare – the antithyroid drug may prevent the bone marrow from working properly. The white corpuscles in the blood are manufactured in the bone marrow, and in agranulocytosis the white cells, known as granulocytes, are reduced in number or completely disappear from the blood. These cells are normally very active in fighting off micro-organisms that may invade the body. Usually the first symptom of agranulocytosis is a sore throat due to micro-organisms invading the tonsillar area at the back of the mouth. Thus every patient taking antithyroid drugs must know that if a sore throat develops, the antithyroid drug must be stopped and the patient should within 12 hours go to their doctor or hospital to have a white cell count done. If this shows that the white corpuscles (the granulocytes) are very depleted, penicillin is usually given to kill off the invading organisms until such time as the marrow has recovered and the white cells have returned to the bloodstream in the normal numbers. In the past an attempt was sometimes made to anticipate the development of agranulocytosis by doing a white cell count every month during treatment. This gave a false sense of security because agranulocytosis may develop suddenly: the white cell count may be normal one day and agranulocytosis develop 3–4 days later. Thus it is safer if the patient is forewarned, without being frightened, and knows to stop treatment and report if a sore throat develops.

Subtotal thyroidectomy

Surgical removal of most of the thyroid gland is a very effective treatment for Graves' disease. When hyperthyroidism is due to multinodular toxic goitre or a toxic adenoma, this can be treated by surgical excision or by radio-iodine. Before operation the hyperthyroid patient must be rendered euthyroid either with Lugol's iodine or an antithyroid drug or both.

In the hands of an experienced thyroid surgeon and a skilled anaesthetist the patient is seldom in hospital for more than 5–7 days. Although the quality of the scar can never be guaranteed in most instances it is almost invisible a year after the operation. The incision in the skin is made across the neck usually in one of the natural creases already there. Techniques from plastic surgery are used to close the wound after some seven-eighths of the thyroid gland has been removed. Most surgeons tend deliberately to remove rather too much of the gland rather than too little. This is to prevent leaving too much gland with the risk of the remnant being sufficiently large to allow a recurrence of hyperthyroidism. If this does happen a second operation, though possible, is best avoided because second operations are followed by an increased incidence of complications. If there is a recurrence, a small dose of radio-iodine is usually used in patients of any age or sex to cure the thyrotoxicosis.

Surgical treatment is mainly used in patients aged 18–40 and in older patients with hyperthyroidism associated with a cosmetically unsightly goitre. It is also the preferred treatment in most patients with a toxic retrosternal goitre particularly if this is of sufficient size to be distorting or compressing the windpipe. If the windpipe is severely compressed the patient may experience some difficulty in breathing, but before this happens they often when asleep make a curious crowing noise. This stridor occurs as the patient's head slumps forwards or to one side when they are fast asleep, and the relaxed neck muscles allow the thyroid gland to compress the trachea even more. In this type of disorder treatment with antithyroid drugs for a prolonged period or with radio-iodine should generally be avoided because either of these treatments may temporarily increase the size of the goitre and aggravate the degree of windpipe compression.

In a variable proportion of patients — around 20 per cent — whose thyrotoxicosis is treated surgically, underactivity of the thyroid gland develops post-operatively. The surgeon cannot be blamed for this because he may rightly have veered towards removing too much rather than too little of the gland. After the operation the patient must be kept under observation and if hypothyroidism is going to develop as a direct consequence of surgery this is usually obvious within three months on clinical grounds confirmed by laboratory tests (Chapter 7). Hypothyroidism may also develop later because of autoimmune destruction of the thyroid remnant and this occurs more commonly in patients whose blood contains pre-operatively a high level of microsomal antibodies. If underactivity does develop this is easily treated by giving thyroxine to make good the deficit.

Two other complications may follow subtotal thyroidectomy. Running in or near the thyroid gland are on the right and left side of the neck nerves that activate the vocal cords. If these nerves are bruised the patient may have a hoarse voice post-operatively, although often huskiness of the voice for a day or so is the consequence of the anaesthetic. Permanent hoarseness of the voice will occur if one of the nerves to the vocal cords is actually cut, but this seldom if ever happens with an experienced thyroid surgeon using modern techniques.

The other possible post-operative complication of subtotal thyroidectomy is related to the parathyroid glands. Usually there are four of these pea-sized glands (two on each side) which lie towards the back of the thyroid gland and may be embedded in it. The surgeon makes every endeavour not to remove these parathyroid glands and it is most uncommon for all four to be lost. But they may be bruised during the operation and therefore may not function properly for some days or even weeks afterwards. The parathyroid glands regulate the level of calcium in the bloodstream. If they do not function properly the level of calcium falls and this may give rise to a clinical condition called tetany. In this the patient tends to be rather upset emotionally. The first physical symptom is usually numbness of the lips and round the mouth. Later the patient may experience cramp in the hands and sometimes in the feet. These symptoms can be corrected by giving the patient calcium with or without vitamin D to restore the blood calcium level to normal. Usually such treatment is only necessary for a short time but very occasionally it is required permanently.

Thyroid disease: the facts

Radio-iodine treatment

In many respects this is a very convenient form of treatment for Graves' disease, a multinodular toxic goitre or a toxic adenoma. The radio-iodine is taken by mouth through a straw It tastes like water and is administered on an out-patient basis. There is no operation, no scar, no anaesthetic, and no significant time off work. The amount of radio-iodine given varies according to whether the patient has a multinodular toxic goitre, a toxic adenoma, or Graves' disease, and if the last according to the size of the thyroid gland and the degree of its overactivity. Although this treatment has an early effect on the making of T_4 and T_3 by the thyroid cells, its maximum effect is not achieved until three months have passed. During this time it is often possible to keep the patient comfortable by suppressing their thyrotoxic symptoms with a beta-blocking drug such as propranolol. In very severe cases antithyroid drugs are given until the radio-iodine has produced its maximum beneficial effect. Radio-iodine has been used in the treatment of hyperthyroidism for 40 years and has proved itself a safe form of treatment. Because of possible genetic effects from radiation to the ovaries or testes, this treatment is in the United Kingdom seldom given to patients aged less than 40, although in the United States it may be used in patients as young as 18 or 20. Despite the theoretical genetic risks, radio-iodine is used in the younger patient who has relapsed after subtotal thyroidectomy because radio-iodine is safer than a second operation which is more likely than the first to result in damage to the nerves supplying the vocal cords or to the parathyroid glands.

Radio-iodine is never given to a hyperthyroid pregnant woman because from the third month onwards the thyroid gland of the fetus can take up iodine and would therefore be irradiated.

The major disadvantage, which must be weighed against

the many advantages, of radio-iodine in the treatment of Graves' disease is the liability for hypothyroidism to develop sooner or later during the next 20 years. This happens in Graves' disease because the whole gland is initially overactive and hence the whole gland is irradiated. The position with a toxic adenoma is rather different because only the adenoma is active and the radioactive material is concentrated in this area with sparing of the remainder of the gland. Something of the order of half the patients with Graves' disease develop hypothyroidism after ^{131}I treatment and the incidence is not materially influenced by the dose of radio-iodine given. Provided the patient is kept under annual observation the hazard of developing hypothyroidism is negligible, because replacement therapy with thyroxine by mouth can be started as soon as evidence of thyroid deficiency appears. In this sort of case keeping the patient under annual observation can mean seeing the doctor once a year, or answering a postal questionnaire every year, and then having a blood test if the answers to the questionnaire merit it, or having a blood test done annually. Probably the ideal is to see the doctor and have a blood test annually.

Treatment of the eye complications

This is never easy; it requires patience and tolerance on the part of the patient and much understanding on the part of the doctor, who has to combine, because the cause of the eye complications is ill-understood, intuitive art, experience, and science in helping the patient. If the condition of the eyes is stable or improving, little or no treatment may be necessary. If the patient is a man, in the older age group over 50, or the patient has developed ophthalmopathy soon after subtotal thyroidectomy or treatment with radio-iodine, a very careful watch must be kept because in these situations there is an increased risk of the eye complications becoming progressively worse. When the ophthalmopathy is progressing active treatment is called for.

Lid retraction and lid lag. Retraction of the upper eyelid may respond to treatment with propranolol with a reduction in the stariness of the eyes. Sometimes drops of guanethidine instilled into the eyes prove helpful, but often the patient complains that the drops even in half-strength cause a stinging discomfort. The main encouragement is that as the hyperthyroidism comes under control, with whatever form of treatment is used, the stariness diminishes in two-thirds of patients. The less the forward bulging of the eyeballs (proptosis or exophthalmos) the less likely is the lid retraction to be permanent, particularly if treatment is started early. When the lid retraction and lid lag are of long-standing and scar-tissue (fibrosis) has developed in the upper lids, surgery may be used to lower the position of the lids.

Exophthalmos. Infiltrative ophthalmopathy may be a more serious and difficult problem, depending on its severity and its progression. In any one individual case it is hard to predict the outcome. As the hyperthyroidism is brought and kept under control or cured, lessening of the exophthalmos occurs spontaneously in 5–10 per cent of patients, but this is often a slow improvement occurring almost imperceptibly over many years. In about three-quarters the exophthalmos remains static unless special measures are taken and a good response to medical treatment, as opposed to surgical treatment, cannot be guaranteed. In 15–20 per cent of patients the infiltrative ophthalmopathy worsens and this is more common in men, particularly the older ones, and perhaps also when radio-iodine is used for treatment of the hyperthyroidism.

Protrusion of one or both eyes is cosmetically unsightly. Because the protruding eye is less well covered and lubricated by the eyelids, the front of the eye (the cornea) is more prone to injury by wind, dust, and infection. Drops of artificial tears may relieve the feeling of grittiness. In more severe cases corticosteroid eye drops may be helpful and

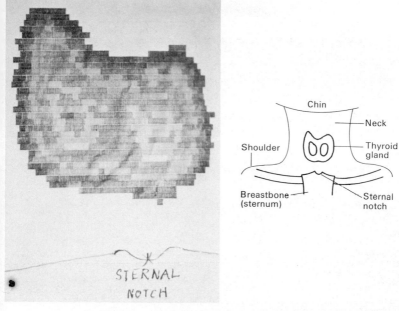

Plate 1. Normal technetium isotope scan of the thyroid gland. The outline of the gland is clearly shown. The right lobe is slightly larger than the left. The degree of uptake of the isotope is greatest in the centre of each lobe where there is the most thyroid tissue. The 'sternal notch' is the small hollow at the upper end of the breast-bone.

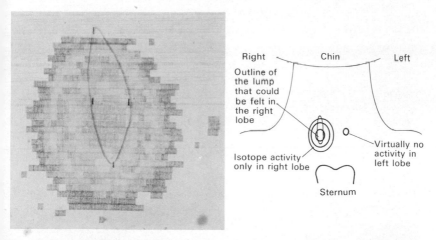

Plate 2. Technetium isotope scan of a thyroid gland containing a toxic adenoma. The 'hot' nodule in the right lobe takes up all the isotope, and there is virtually no radioactivity in the other lobe because it is inactive as a result of T_4 from the nodule suppressing the secretion of TSH from the pituitary gland (see text).

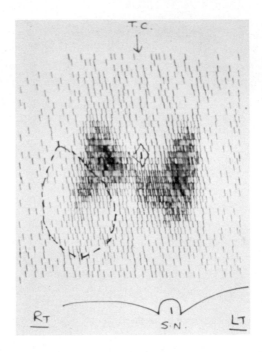

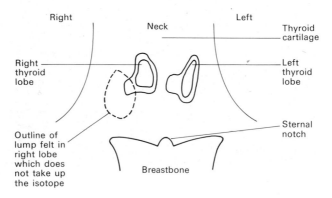

Plate 3. Technetium scan of the thyroid gland containing a 'cold' nodule. The outline of the nodule in the lower part of the right lobe, which could easily be seen and felt, has been inked in on the scan. There is no radioactivity in this nodule which is therefore 'cold'.

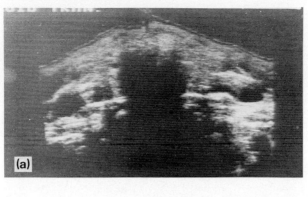

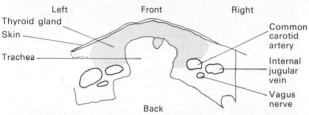

Left   Front   Right

Thyroid gland

Skin

Trachea

Common carotid artery

Internal jugular vein

Vagus nerve

Back

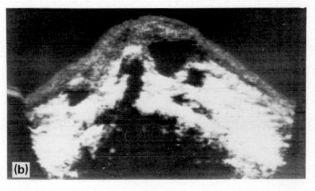

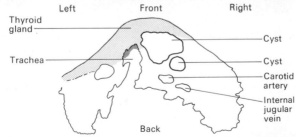

Left   Front   Right

Thyroid gland

Trachea

Cyst

Cyst

Carotid artery

Internal jugular vein

Back

Plate 4. Ultrasound scans of the thyroid gland. (a) Normal. (b) A large and a small cyst in the right lobe are causing some thyroid enlargement.

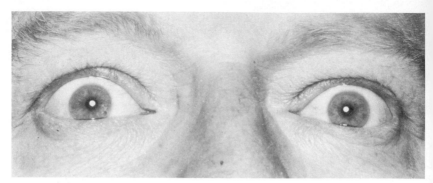

Plate 5. Lid retraction. Note how the upper eyelids are retracted so that the eyes have a staring quality and more of the white of the eyes than normal is visible.

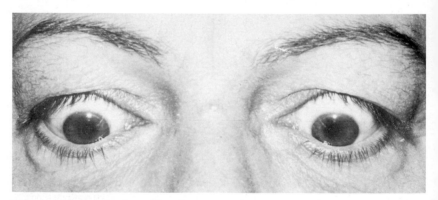

Plate 6. Lid lag. As the patient looks downwards, the upper lid lags behind the eyeball.

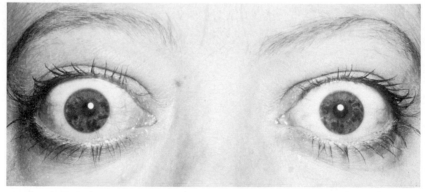

Plate 7. Exophthalmos or proptosis. Both eyeballs are more prominent than normal and protrude forwards. There is some swelling of the soft tissues above the upper eyelids. Note also the eyes are somewhat bloodshot, the right more than the left.

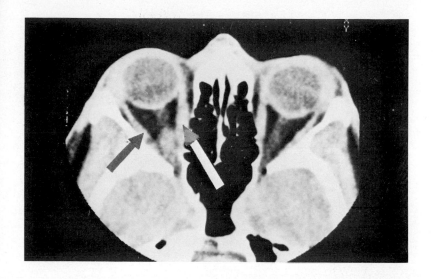

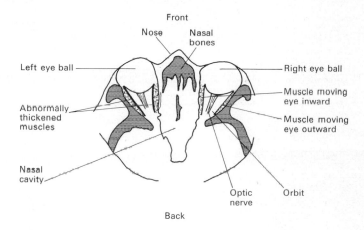

Front

Nose Nasal
bones

Left eye ball

Right eye ball

Muscle moving
eye inward

Abnormally
thickened
muscles

Muscle moving
eye outward

Nasal
cavity

Optic
nerve

Orbit

Back

Plate 8. Computerized tomographic (CT) or computer-assisted tomographic (CAT) scan of the orbits, taken from above, in a patient with impaired movements of the left eye, ophthalmoplegia, and double vision when looking up-wards and to the left (diplopia). The eyeballs can be clearly seen, and some of the muscles (marked with an arrow) that move the left eyeball are thicker than those in the right orbit.

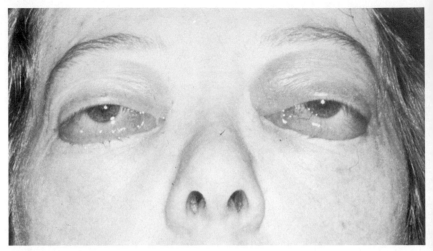

Plate 9. Severe ophthalmopathy in Graves' disease before treatment. The eyeballs are protruding forwards but the extent of this exophthalmos is in part masked by the swelling in and around the eyelids.

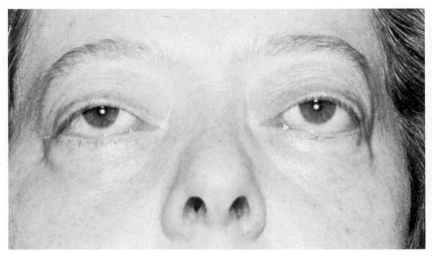

Plate 10. Ten days after treatment with prednisone (a corticosteroid drug) the ophthalmopathy (shown in Plate 9) is much improved. The eyes are less 'angry' and uncomfortable. The swelling of the eyelids is much reduced but upward movement of the eyeballs is still defective, which explains why the patient holds her head tilted back.

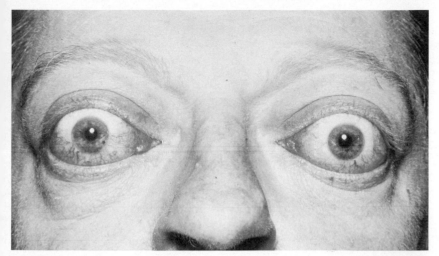

Plate 11. Marked ophthalmopathy showing exophthalmos, lid retraction, and redness of the scleral blood vessels.

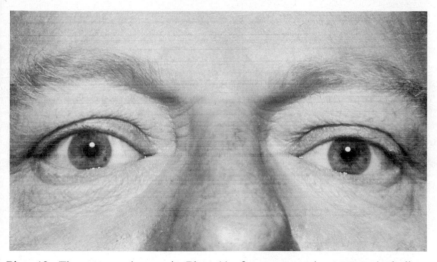

Plate 12. The same patient as in Plate 11 after two years' treatment including decompression of both orbits.

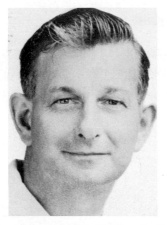
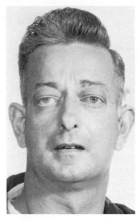

Plate 13. Appearance before (left) and after (right) the development of thyrotoxicosis.

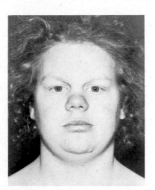
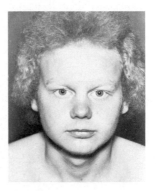

Plate 14. A 17-year-old carpenter with myxoedema (hypothyroidism) (left) before treatment; (right) after 18 months' treatment with thyroxine.

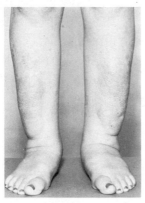
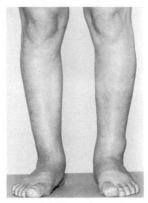

Plate 15. Pretibial myxoedema: (left) before treatment and (right) the appearance of the legs 18 months after treatment with thyroxine by mouth and the local application of corticosteroid ointment.

antibiotic eye drops or ointment may be required if there is infection of the cornea. Some protection is provided by dark glasses with side pieces that protect the eyeballs from wind and dust blowing in from the side. Swelling of the soft tissues above the upper eyelids and below the lower lids may be reduced by having the patient sleep propped up on high pillows and taking a diuretic which increases the elimination of water from the body.

When the degree of exophthalmos is more extreme, the outer one-quarter or less of the eyelids can under local anaesthetic be temporarily or permanently sewn together (tarsorrhaphy). This narrows the opening between the upper and lower lids and provides better coverage of, and protection to, the eyeballs. This operation may also be used to improve the patient's cosmetic appearance because it reduces the stariness of the eyes and the apparent protrusion of the eyeballs.

When the protrusion of the eyeballs is progressive, cortisone-like drugs (corticosteroids) can be effective (Plates 9 and 10). Later when the acute phase is over, surgical enlargement of the bony orbit will allow the increased orbital tissue to expand in another direction so that the degree of ocular protrusion is substantially reduced. Various operations to achieve this have been devised but in the most modern the floor of the orbit is removed from inside the mouth without making any externally visible scar. The improvement, both from the point of view of ocular discomfort and cosmetic appearance, can be striking (Plates 11 and 12).

Ophthalmoplegia and double vision. Infiltration of the oculomotor muscles that move the eyeballs impairs their action so that the eyes cease to be parallel to each other. Scarring or fibrosis of the muscles at the bottom of the eyes prevents the patient from being able to look upwards. Inflammation followed by fibrosis of the inner muscles prevents the eyes from being moved outwards. The results of these impaired movements (ophthalmoplegia) is double vision (diplopia).

This disability tends to improve in two-thirds of patients when their hyperthyroidism is brought under control but a favourable response cannot be guaranteed and at best any improvement is slow. The double vision is a major problem to the patient. During the acute initial phase reading or watching television is made more tolerable by wearing a patch over one eye or, if the patient wears spectacles, painting nail varnish over the inside of one lens so that the patient has only monocular vision and sees only one image. Glass prisms can be used or fitted to existing spectacles to correct the diplopia and allow safe driving of a car. Corticosteroid treatment may prove helpful. When the condition of the eyes is static and the acute ophthalmopathy is quiescent and 'burnt out', definitive surgical adjustment of the oculomotor muscles can be carried out to correct the double vision permanently. This should not be done until after orbital decompression has been carried out, if this is planned, to correct severe exophthalmos.

Malignant exophthalmos. When infiltrative ophthalmopathy is progressive and severe, there is protrusion of the eyes, swelling of the soft tissues above the upper lids and below the lower lids, irritation of the exposed surface of the eye, and double vision. The eyes look red and angry. They water excessively and the patient experiences grittiness and severe discomfort. In some instances infection of the eye as a whole occurs, or there may be a progressive deterioration in vision. Treatment with cortisone-like drugs (corticosteroids) can have a dramatically beneficial effect. Plate 9 shows acute ophthalmopathy due to Graves' disease, and Plate 10 the response 10 days later to prednisone treatment. This form of treatment given at the appropriate time and sometimes in conjunction with other drugs, such as azathioprine (Imuran), that reduce the immunological reaction in the orbit can be very helpful. Such treatment may also be of great value when the increased pressure in the orbit threatens the patient's vision by compressing the optic nerve which carries the light signals from the eye to that part of the brain where the signals are interpreted.

When the response to corticosteroid treatment is incomplete, and particularly if vision is threatened, surgical measures may be required to reduce the increased pressure within the bony orbit.

Treatment of pretibial myxoedema

The course of pretibial myxoedema is unpredictable. Almost invariably it is associated with ophthalmopathy of severe degree and these eye complications may be of more concern to the patient. As the patient's hyperthyroidism responds to treatment so the pretibial myxoedema may remit, particularly if cortisone-like drugs are used to treat the ophthalmopathy.

Pretibial myxoedema may however not become apparent until the patient's thyrotoxicosis has been cured. Thus, like the eye complications, pretibial myxoedema may precede hyperthyroidism, develop concurrently with thyrotoxicosis, or develop after thyroid overactivity has been cured. The most effective treatment is to apply a very potent corticosteroid ointment each night to the affected area on the leg, rub it well in, and then wrap round the involved part of the leg a layer of polythene film such as is used in the kitchen for covering open dishes or to preserve vegetables in a refrigerator. This treatment may have to be continued over a prolonged period of time.

5

Subacute viral thyroiditis

This condition, also known as de Quervain's thyroiditis after a Swiss physician who first described the clinical features, is a relatively rare thyroid disorder. Although uncommon in the United Kingdom or other parts of Europe, it seems to be more common in North America. Because the disease tends to run a self-limiting course, mild cases may never be seen by a doctor and there can be no doubt that even in more severe cases the correct diagnosis is often missed.

The condition occurs more often in women than men and it seems that those with a pre-existing small goitre are most vulnerable. Many different viruses are capable of causing thyroiditis, the most prevalent being the Coxsackie (a virus first isolated in a small township in New York State) and the mumps viruses. Except for research purposes, attempts to isolate the offending virus are seldom made because the techniques are difficult and expensive, and even if the precise virus is identified we do not yet have effective antibiotics to kill it.

Typical clinical picture

The illness starts with a non-specific malaise characterized by tiredness, muscular aches and pains of no great severity, and sometimes a mild headache. There may be a slight fever up to 37.2–37.8°C (99–100°F). After a few days of this 'flu-like illness there is discomfort in the region of the thyroid gland. Often the patient gently rubs the front of the neck. Swallowing becomes painful, and characteristically stabs of pain or an ache may run upwards from the front of the neck to the ear on one or both sides. The thyroid gland has now been invaded by the virus and becomes inflamed and tender to the touch. The degree of enlargement is slight.

Because the thyroid is inflamed, the hormones leach out and the blood levels of T_4 and T_3 rise. The patient becomes mildly thyrotoxic, with an increased heart rate, nervousness, tremor, sweating, and often a minor degree of weight loss. The thyrotoxic features may not be prominent, and many patients who seek medical advice go to their doctor complaining of a 'sore throat' and some discomfort each time they swallow. Unless the patient makes it clear that the soreness is truly in the front of the neck, which is after all the throat, the doctor may focus his attention on the throat at the back of the mouth, and find that the tonsillar area is normal or only slightly pink. Unless he perceives that it is the thyroid gland which is tender, the diagnosis will be missed.

Many cases of subacute viral thyroiditis run a self-limiting course over 3–6 weeks, and a stoical patient may ignore the symptoms. More severe cases last longer, wax and wane in severity, and make the patient feel quite ill. In others the condition is relatively painless, and the mild thyrotoxic symptoms dominate the clinical picture; this seems particularly common in North America.

Diagnosis

Often the diagnosis can be made from the patient's characteristic story and the finding of a tender slightly enlarged thyroid gland. Provided the condition is suspected, the diagnosis can readily be confirmed if the right tests are carried out. During the acute inflammatory phase the blood level of thyroid hormones (T_4 and/or T_3) is raised, but this occurs in other patients with hyperthyroidism irrespective of the cause. In subacute viral thyroiditis the function of the thyroid cells is so deranged by the inflammation that the gland does not take up iodine from the bloodstream. Thus a radioactive thyroid scan with radio-iodine or technetium will show little or no uptake. With reference to the analogy of the car factory in Chapter 3 (p. 15), this is a situation when no raw steel is going into the factory yet more than the normal number of finished cars are coming out at the other end. The combination of high T_4 and T_3 levels and no uptake of isotope by the gland is virtually diagnostic of de Quervain's thyroiditis. However similar laboratory results occur in a patient who, often secretly, is taking an excessive number of thyroxine tablets, but in such a case the gland is not tender and there is no discomfort in the throat.

Sometimes it is necessary to distinguish subacute viral thyroiditis from the early stages of Hashimoto's thyroiditis (Chapter 6), when there may be some discomfort in the thyroid associated with mild hyperthyroidism ('Hashi-toxicosis'). In this condition the thyroid uptake of isotope is at this stage normal or increased and the key to the diagnosis is the high level of thyroid auto-antibodies in the bloodstream — levels that are much higher than the zero or low amounts found in de Quervain's thyroid-itis.

Treatment

Mild cases of de Quervain's thyroiditis may need no treatment, or the discomfort in the neck can be made less with aspirin or paracetamol. When the condition is more severe, two drugs in combination will greatly help the patient. Propranolol is used to mitigate the symptoms caused by the hyperthyroidism (see Chapter 4, p. 44). Prednisone, a cortisone-like compound, reduces the acute inflammatory changes in the thyroid gland and is necessary when the pain is severe. The usual practice is to give a fairly large dose (30–40 mg daily) for the first week and then gradually to reduce the dosage over the next three weeks. Sometimes the condition relapses and the course of corticosteroids has to be repeated.

Subacute viral thyroiditis

It is very unusual for viral thyroiditis to damage the thyroid gland permanently, but occasionally hypothyroidism develops later.

6

Hashimoto's thyroiditis

Hashimoto's or autoimmune thyroiditis is for several reasons an important disease. (1) It is a significant cause of goitre in children aged 10 or over and even more so in adults, with a marked preponderance for women — the female to male ratio being 10 or even 20 to 1. The goitre is seldom large. (2) Hashimoto's thyroiditis is an important cause of hypothyroidism. In many parts of the world it is the most common cause of thyroid deficiency though in others lack of dietary iodine (p. 69) ranks first. (3) Hashimoto's thyroiditis was one of the first autoimmune diseases in medicine to be recognized, and its understanding has thrown light on other autoimmune disorders. We still do not know why certain white corpuscles (lymphocytes) come to regard thyroid tissue as 'foreign' (Chapter 2), but these lymphocytes with their associated thyroid antibodies attack the thyroid gland and gradually destroy it.

Course of the disease

The course of the disease is usually protracted over many years, and during this time waxes and wanes in its destructive effect on the thyroid gland. At any stage the disease may become arrested or appear to lie dormant. The patient may present to the doctor different symptoms depending on the stage to which the disease has progressed. Most will seek advice in the later phases when hypothyroidism has developed, but let us follow an imaginary patient along the road of untreated Hashimoto's thyroiditis.

At the age of 18, or earlier, the patient's parents may first notice slight enlargement of their daughter's thyroid gland.

Hashimoto's thyroiditis

Over the next two years it increases slightly in size and becomes obvious to the practised eye. The gland is enlarged because there is some increase in the jelly-like colloid (thyroglobulin) and because the gland is infiltrated with lymphocytes and related autoimmune cells. At this stage the gland will feel quite soft and fleshy, and the patient's blood will contain thyroid antibodies in small or moderate amounts. The patient will feel perfectly well.

At the age of 28 the gland may be slightly less large. For some weeks or months the patient may experience intermittently discomfort in the front of her throat and on occasions swallowing may be slightly painful. The lymphocytes are continuing their attack on the thyroid tissue and the inflammatory reaction may be sufficiently intense to cause the discomfort in the neck and slight tenderness on pressing the gland. The gland will now feel firmer, and because of the lymphocyte infiltration is in some countries called a lymphadenoid goitre.

A small proportion of patients with Hashimoto's thyroiditis experience for a few weeks or months mild symptoms of hyperthyroidism — so-called 'Hashitoxicosis'. Very occasionally such patients develop slight eye complications of the type seen in Graves' disease (p. 38). The Hashitoxicosis may be due to T_4 and T_3 being leached out of the gland by the inflammatory reaction or, more probably, it is due to the transient development of thyroid-stimulating antibodies in addition to the microsomal and thyroglobulin antibodies associated with thyroid destruction.

Later at the age of 48 after a period of inactivity — a truce — the destructive process resumes. The gland may now have difficulty in manufacturing adequate amounts of T_4 and T_3. As a result of the feedback mechanism (Chapter 1), the pituitary secretion of TSH rises in an attempt to drive the flagging thyroid gland to increased activity. At this stage the gland seldom becomes more prominent in response to the increased secretion of TSH because little normal thyroid tissue is left and the gland is scarred (fibrosed) by the previous inflammatory reaction induced by the invading lymphocytes. At this time the level of microsomal and/or thyroglobulin antibodies is usually high.

Finally at the age of 58 the gland is destroyed. No longer is sufficient thyroid tissue left to make adequate amounts of T_4 and T_3, and the patient becomes hypothyroid. At this last stage the gland may be slightly enlarged, normal in size, or so shrunken and fibrosed that it can no longer be felt. If the gland can be felt, it is harder than normal. Sometimes one or two nodules may be discernible and these usually represent small areas of normal thyroid tissue which have escaped the inflammatory attack but are insufficient in amount to sustain euthyroidism.

Few patients with Hashimoto's thyroiditis will consciously experience all these stages, and fewer doctors will be in practice long enough to follow such a patient over 40 years.

Diagnosis

Essentially the diagnosis of autoimmune thyroiditis is based on the finding of high levels of microsomal and/or thyro-globulin antibodies in the patient's blood, levels which to a certain point increase as the disease progresses. In the last phases of the disease when all the thyroid tissue has been destroyed, the stimulus to antibody formation may have been eliminated, and the level of thyroid microsomal and/or thyroglobulin auto-antibodies may fall to low or undetectable levels, thus making it hard to be sure why the patient has developed thyroid failure.

Thyroid secretory function must be monitored throughout the long course of Hashimoto's thyroiditis because it is this which determines the patient's well-being. Certainly treatment with thyroxine will often reduce the size of the goitre in most cases at any stage, but this therapy will be particularly necessary when the T_4 or T_3 level falls below normal (Chapter

7). Some doctors find it logical to start treatment with T_4 when there is evidence of impending thyroid failure as shown by a low normal T_4 level but a TSH raised above 20 mU/l. Those who hold this view point out that sooner or later the patient may become hypothyroid and this is best prevented by starting replacement therapy earlier rather than later.

Treatment

We have no safe reliable way of modifying the faulty immunological surveillance whereby lymphocytes mistakenly judge thyroid tissue to be 'foreign'. There are drugs (corticosteroids and immuno-suppressants) which reduce immunological rejection but such agents are mainly used in life-threatening situations such as the rejection of a donated kidney. Hashimoto's thyroiditis is not a life-threatening disease and the use of potentially dangerous therapy is not justified. Furthermore this treatment might have to be continued indefinitely. Thus the basic cause of Hashimoto's thyroiditis is not treated.

If there is a short-lived phase of Hashitoxicosis, propranolol or an antithyroid drug, such as carbimazole, may be given for a time (p. 44 and 48). If the gland becomes painful a short course of corticosteroids may be used as in subacute viral thyroiditis (p. 60).

In general the treatment of Hashimoto's thyroiditis is the management of its hypothyroid consequences, although an unsightly goitre can usually be reduced in size by giving thyroxine. The essential measure is the prevention of hypothyroidism when this is imminent or the correction of hypothyroidism when this has developed. Thus the treatment is replacement therapy with thyroxine (p. 75).

Occasionally surgery is required, particularly if there is any possibility that the goitre is due to cancer and not Hashimoto's thyroiditis. This differential difficulty arises when the thyroid feels very hard or is enlarged asymmetrically.

Surgery is also advisable if there is hoarseness of the voice, symptoms due to compression of the windpipe, or the goitre is cosmetically unsightly despite treatment with thyroxine.

Associated diseases

Hashimoto's thyroiditis may be associated with other auto-immune disorders. Some 10 per cent of patients with Hashimoto's thyroiditis may develop Addisonian (formerly called pernicious) anaemia (p. 30). Others develop diabetes, but this is rare. Some patients, perhaps 5 per cent, have associated polymyalgia rheumatica, a disorder characterized by muscular pains and weakness. Very rarely autoimmune destruction of the parathyroid or adrenal glands or of the ovaries or testes may occur. Lack of secretion of tears and saliva (Sjörgren's syndrome) is an occasional accompaniment as may be the gradual appearance of areas of unusually white depigmented skin (vitiligo or leucoderma).

7

Hypothyroidism

Hypothyroidism is the clinical condition that develops when there is inadequate secretion of thyroxine (T_4) and triiodothyronine (T_3) by the thyroid gland. Irrespective of the cause of the thyroid deficiency, the symptoms and clinical picture in the adult are the same although these vary in their severity according to the degree of the deficiency and its duration. Myxoedema is the word used to describe advanced hypothyroidism.

Hypothyroidism should be looked upon as a graded phenomenon with a continuous range starting with slightly diminished thyroid function, only revealed by sophisticated laboratory tests, and progressing to complete thyroid failure that is clinically obvious and associated with unequivocally abnormal laboratory findings (Table 5).

Hypothyroidism may occur at any age but is most common in women between the ages of 30 and 60. It may occur in infants (cretinism) and in older children (juvenile myxoedema); in both these groups the clinical picture is rather different from that in adults, from which it will be considered separately.

Causes of adult hypothyroidism

There are many causes of deficient thyroid secretion. Two obvious ones are removal of too much thyroid tissue during subtotal thyroidectomy in the surgical treatment of hyper-thyroidism and destruction of too much of the gland in the treatment of hyperthyroidism with radioactive iodine.

In the Western world Hashimoto's thyroiditis is the commonest cause of 'spontaneous' hypothyroidism and is the presumed cause of thyroid failure in patients who have

Table 5 *The grading of thyroid failure*

Grade	Symptoms of hypothyroidism	T_4	T_3	Basal TSH	TRH test
Very early impairment	None	Normal	Normal	Normal	Abnormal increase of TSH at 20 min.
Compensated impairment	None	Normal	Normal (rarely a little raised)	Slightly raised	Abnormal increase
Occult or mild hypothyroidism	None or mild	Slightly low	Normal or slightly low	Raised	Abnormal increase
Overt hypothyroidism	Mild or marked	Low	Low	Very raised	Abnormal increase

Hypothyroidism

shrunken glands even though the level of microsomal thyroid antibodies is no longer raised (p. 64). The prevalence of hypothyroidism is substantial. In the general population about 1.5 women per 100 have overt hypothyroidism but in men the incidence is much lower being less than 0.1 per cent. Lesser degrees of mild or subclinical hypothyroidism (Table 5) with a raised basal TSH level and thyroid antibodies occur in about 3 per cent of the overall population and an even higher prevalence in women aged 50 or more.

In some parts of the world iodine deficiency is the most common cause of thyroid failure. Lack of iodine precludes the thyroid from having enough raw material to manufacture T_4 and T_3. This example of trying to make bricks without straw is usually associated with a sizeable goitre, whereas in the conditions mentioned earlier little or no thyroid tissue can usually be felt.

There are other less common, and therefore less important, causes of hypothyroidism. Certain drugs, such as the anti-thyroid drugs used to control hyperthyroidism (p. 45) will reduce the production of T_4 and T_3 below normal if given in too large a dose for too long. Some patients are 'sensitive' to medicines which contain iodides such as over-the-counter cough and asthma cures and become hypothyroid with prolonged self-treatment. Lithium is used for the treatment of certain mental disorders; in susceptible subjects it may depress thyroid function but of this psychiatrists are well aware. Certain foods, such as cabbage, other 'greens' related to kale (notably in Tasmania), and seaweed (particularly in Japan), contain anti-thyroid compounds.

Clinical picture in adults

The severity of the symptoms in hypothyroidism depend upon the degree of thyroid failure and upon its rate of onset. In most instances of 'spontaneous' thyroid failure overt hypothyroidism creeps up on the patient. The changes are so imperceptibly slow in their development that for some long time they are seldom recognized by either the patient or those closest to her. 'Her' is used because the disease is ten times more common in women than in men.

Overt hypothyroidism. Lethargy is the first manifestation. Intolerance of cold is another early feature. The patient wants more domestic heating later in the spring or earlier in the autumn; she wears thicker clothing when the rest of the family are lightly clad. Menstruation may be heavier and more prolonged. Some gain in weight is common but seldom more than 10 lb (4 kg) over a year. The skin becomes dry and the scalp hair may be lost at an increased rate. The eyebrows thin, and hair on the forearms becomes short and stubbly. Axillary and pubic hair may become scanty. The hands are podgy. The voice becomes deeper in pitch. Hearing is dulled so that the patient is the last in the family to hear the telephone ring. Normal bowel function is replaced by constipation. Muscular aches and pains are common. The patient may become unsteady on her feet (ataxia), fall, and then with loss of confidence refuse to venture out of the home.

In severe untreated cases changes occur in the patient's physical appearance, speech, and mental attitude. Words become less well articulated so that speech is hoarse, slowed, and slurred like a drunk. The patient's face becomes puffy and lugubrious. The skin has a yellow tinge although the cheeks may remain surprisingly pink. The eyelids and hands are puffy. The patient may complain of pins and needles in the fingers and hands particularly on waking in the morning (carpal tunnel syndrome). There may be swelling of the ankles; the patient is bloated. Her movements are slow and her thought processes are retarded. Rarely psychological changes develop. The patient may become depressed or develop 'myxoedema madness' in which she hears voices, believes that her food is being poisoned, and becomes agitated.

70

Hypothyroidism

These changes are the consequence of a slowing up in the metabolism of all cells in all parts of the body. To the doctor, to whom the patient's appearance may be diagnostic at first sight, these changes are reflected in slowing of the patient's pulse and in sluggishness of the tendon reflexes to relax (p. 14). Fluid retention with associated shortness of breath may be characterized by ankle swelling and the collection of 'water' in the abdominal cavity (ascites), in the thorax around the lungs (pleural effusion), or around the heart (pericardial effusion).

Changes in the metabolism of fats, notably cholesterol, occur. The resulting high cholesterol level is associated with accelerated narrowing of the arteries (atheroma). Some elevation of blood pressure is common. On walking, particularly fast or up an incline, the patient may experience tight constricting pain across the chest (angina pectoris) due to narrowing of the coronary arteries to the heart's muscle, or a cramp in the calves due to narrowing of the arteries carrying blood to the legs (intermittent claudication). Either may compel the patient to stop walking and rest.

Rarely, in neglected cases, the patient lapses into myxoedema coma. This often fatal complication only occurs in severe cases, usually in cold weather and in women who live alone, unvisited by friends or relatives.

Mild hypothyroidism. Lesser degrees of hypothyroidism may occur (Table 5) and can be difficult to diagnose, because the symptoms are often vague and non-specific. The possibility of mild thyroid failure will be entertained in anyone who for no evident reason — physical or emotional — complains of tiredness, heavy menstrual loss (which may of course induce tiredness by rendering the patient anaemic), cold intolerance, bloatedness, dryness of the skin, constipation of recent origin, or hair loss. Particularly should hypothyroidism be considered if there is a family history of any sort of thyroid disease or of pernicious anaemia, or if the patient has vitiligo (p. 66).

71

Diagnosis of adult hypothyroidism

In clinically obvious hypothyroidism, the T_4 and T_3 levels are depressed far below the lower end of the normal range. The TSH level is raised often being in excess of 100 mU/l. In milder and earlier cases the T_4 level may be near or only just below the lower limits of the normal range. The T_3 level may be normal or rarely slightly raised but the TSH level, which is the most sensitive indicator of primary thyroid failure, is unequivocally raised (greater than 20 mU/l).

Many indirect tests for detecting hypothyroidism or following its response to treatment have been used. The slowness of the Achilles tendon reflex to relax, the cholesterol level, the elevation of certain muscle (creatine phosphokinase — CPK) and liver (glutamic oxaloacetic [aspartate] transaminase — AST or SGOT) enzymes, which tend to be raised in hypothyroidism, and the electrocardiogram have their uses but are not specific to thyroid dysfunction.

In all cases of overt or suspected hypothyroidism a search should be made for thyroid auto-antibodies, even when the cause of the hypothyroidism is apparently obvious, as for example after thyroid surgery or radio-iodine treatment. This serves as a reminder to the doctor to check for other auto-immune diseases (p. 66). In less obvious or early cases the finding of high levels of thyroid antibodies suggests that thyroid failure may be present and will lead to more sensitive tests of thyroid function being done. A particularly significant combination is a raised TSH and thyroid antibody level. About 5 per cent of women per annum with this combination will develop overt hypothyroidism, and for this reason a good case can be made for starting thyroxine treatment at this stage.

A comparison of the patient's present appearance with earlier photographs may be helpful in suggesting a diagnosis of hypothyroidism, and pictures taken before and after replacement thereapy are often a witness to the striking therapeutic response.

Hypothyroidism

Juvenile myxoedema

The onset of hypothyroidism around the age of 8 years is usually due to improper development of the thyroid gland or less commonly to autoimmune thyroiditis. Up to this time the amount of thyroid tissue in the maldeveloped gland has been adequate to sustain normal T_4 and T_3 levels. As the child grows in size the maldeveloped gland cannot keep pace and hypothyroidism gradually develops. The most prominent and obvious consequence is that the child stops growing. Seldom are there other symptoms and surprisingly the child's intellectual performance at school is usually maintained. Although failure to grow in height is the presenting feature, the patient is often plump and may have pads of fat above the collar-bones. Puberty and sexual development are usually delayed if the condition is left untreated, but occasionally for unknown reasons puberty occurs much earlier than usual.

The diagnosis is based on the same criteria as are used for confirming thyroid failure in an adult. X-rays of the bones will show that their development is retarded in relation to the child's chronological age. An isotope scan of the neck may show slight or no thyroid activity, and in maldevelopment the gland is abnormally small and may be located high in the neck near the root of the tongue (maldescent) instead of in the normal position.

Neonatal hypothyroidism

Thyroid failure in the new-born, if unrecognized, can be disastrous because delay in treatment may result in permanent mental deficiency. In the Western world the most common cause of congenital hypothyroidism is maldevelopment or maldescent of the thyroid gland. The condition has a prevalence of 25–30 cases per 100 000 births. Thus in developed countries every new-born baby is screened biochemically to be sure that it is not thyroid deficient.

Thyroid disease: the facts

In areas of the world where iodine deficiency is common (the Himalayas, the Andes, the Congo region, and New Guinea), the prevalence of neonatal hypothyroidism is even higher and the degree of mental and nervous system damage greater. In these cases the baby's mother usually has a goitre which is mainly due to lack of iodine although other factors such as anti-thyroid substances in the diet may also play a part. This type of endemic neonatal hypothyroidism can be prevented by giving the mother injections of iodized oil or fortifying the salt or bread with iodides.

Clinical picture of congenital hypothyroidism. The features that characterize hypothyroidism in the new-born are often difficult to detect and depend on the degree of thyroid deficiency. They become more obvious as the baby grows older but by then permanent damage to the brain may have occurred. A hypothyroid baby fails to thrive. It does not kick vigorously and sleeps excessively. It is constipated. Its cry may be croaky and the scalp hair may be short and coarse. Often the abdomen is abnormally protuberant; the navel may bulge outwards and be the site of a rupture. The tongue is unusually large and the face to the practised eye has a characteristic flat bloated appearance. Left untreated obvious changes due to involvement of the nervous system — poor co-ordination, tremor, unsteadiness, and excessively brisk reflexes — become apparent. Without biochemical screening half the babies with neonatal hypothyroidism are not diagnosed until they are six months old and cretinism is then established. Although the physical features will disappear with thyroxine replacement thereapy, the mental state may be permanently impaired.

Diagnosis of neonatal hypothyroidism. Every new-born baby should be screened for hypothyroidism on the fifth to tenth day after birth. A needle prick is made in the baby's heel, and four spots of blood placed on a special filter paper card. Two of the blood spots are analysed for TSH, and the other

74

two are used to screen for phenylketonuria (another congenital disease). In hypothyroid babies the TSH level is substantially raised usually to levels in excess of 80 or more mU/l. When the TSH level is 25 to 80 mU/l the test is repeated. Values below 25 mU/l can be regarded as normal. Further confirmation of thyroid deficiency may be obtained by measuring the T_4 concentration but the TSH level is the most reliable and sensitive initial test.

Sometimes congenital hypothyroidism is transient, and without any treatment the baby develops normal thyroid function. This is particularly liable to happen in premature births and in babies of mothers who have been taking thyroid hormones or iodine-containing drugs. It is safer to treat all infants with laboratory evidence of congenital hypothyroidism, and when the baby is about a year old to stop replacement therapy for a few weeks and carefully observe the T_4 and TSH levels. If the T_4 level falls and the TSH rises, replacement therapy must be restarted at once and the baby will not suffer any permanent damage from this temporary withdrawal of treatment. If on the other hand and the T_4 and TSH levels remain normal, the neonatal hypothyroidism was transient.

Treatment of hypothyroidism

The best treatment for hypothyroidism is replacement therapy with thyroxine. Though man-made, medicinal thyroxine is chemically identical to the major hormone secreted by the thyroid gland. Being a pure substance the amount in each tablet can be accurately measured. Three strengths of thyroxine tablets are available — 0.025 mg, 0.05 mg, and 0.1 mg. This is often confusing to the patient particularly as the pharmacist may express the amount of thyroxine in each tablet, not in milligrams (mg = one thousandth of a gram), but as micrograms (μg = one hundred thousandth of a gram) — 25 μg, 50 μg, and 100 μg. Thyroxine is a stable substance and the tablets have a long shelf-life.

Thyroid disease: the facts

The ultimate final dose of thyroxine will depend upon the degree of thyroid failure, and to a lesser extent on the weight and responsiveness of the patient. The total daily dose in an adult with no functioning thyroid tissue at all (a totally athyroid patient) is usually 0.15 to 0.2 mg. Occasionally the dose may need to be 0.25 mg and very rarely 0.3 mg is required.

Thyroxine does not work fast. A tablet taken, for example, on a Monday will induce no biologically discernible effect until the following Friday. Thus the patient need take the thyroxine tablets only once daily and there is no advantage in taking them two or three times a day. Indeed there may be a positive disadvantage in doing this because the patient is liable to forget a dose. Patients have difficulty in remembering even once daily dosage and must learn to take their tablets at a specific time each day. Thus some elect to take the tablets when they clean their teeth or brush their hair on getting up in the morning; others are less likely to forget if they take the tablets when they go to bed each night.

The starting or initial dose of thyroxine will depend upon the degree of hypothyroidism and its duration. If the patient has recently been rendered permanently thyroid deficient by surgery or radio-iodine treatment, no harm will come from starting with 0.1 mg or 0.15 mg and thereafter adjusting the dosage upwards or downwards at six-weekly intervals depending on the patient's clinical response and more importantly on the laboratory results. The aim is to bring the TSH down into the normal range and to maintain the blood thyroxine in the mid- or high normal range.

When hypothyroidism is severe, of long standing, and particularly if the patient has angina the initial dose of thyroxine must be small. Too large a dose given to a patient who has had myxoedema for a year or more is likely to induce palpitations, irregularity of the heart (intermittent due to premature ventricular contractions or more persistent due to atrial fibrillation), shortness of breath, angina, ankle swelling, and heart failure. Particularly in the older patient aged 55 or more too large a starting dose may provoke a constricting pain across the chest on exertion (angina pectoris). Thus in severe long-standing cases of hypothyroidism the initial dose of thyroxine should be 0.025 mg or 0.05 mg daily, and provided no cardiac symptoms are induced the dose is increased every six weeks by increments of 0.025 mg. When the patient is taking a total of 0.1 mg daily (four 0.025 mg tablets or two 0.05 mg tablets), a switch to the stronger 0.1 mg tablets can be made and the final replacement dose determined from the blood levels of T_4 and TSH. All three strengths of tablet are scored so that they can be divided in half with adequate accuracy.

Two problems may arise in the early days of treatment. Some patients experience intermittent and innocent palpitations. A small dose of propranolol (p. 44), 10 to 20 mg twice or three times daily, will usually quell this symptom which is alarming to the patient but not dangerous. Others during the early phases of treatment may experience the 'screws' — muscular aches and pains particularly in the thighs, arms, and back which may make the patient reluctant to increase the dosage of thyroxine or stop treatment altogether. This last will soon become apparent to the doctor who must explain that the muscular pains will pass and that the treatment must be persisted with, and give an analgesic (such as paracetamol or aspirin) to relieve these pains.

The patient must be warned against expecting a miraculous overnight improvement. The longer the duration of the hypothyroidism the longer will it take for the patient to feel really well again — six to nine months in many cases. When the patient has been stabilized on the correct maintenance dose of thyroxine, as judged by a normal TSH level and a serum thyroxine in the upper half of the normal range, it is helpful if a formal note signed and dated by the doctor is given stating the evidence on which the diagnosis of thyroid failure was based, the current replacement therapy and the evidence to show that this is the correct dose of thyroxine. This is necessary because in the years ahead the patient may come under the care of a new doctor, who finding the patient to be well, may doubt the need for continued treatment and stop the thyroxine.

A number of patients receive or self-administer an excessive amount of thyroxine. Most increase the dose themselves initially in the false hope that it will help to lose weight and then persist because the heightened dose increases their energy. There is no doubt that some patients become 'addicted' and take amounts of thyroxine that make them hyperthyroid. One has yet to see the patient who requires more than 0.3 mg thyroxine, and dosages that increase the serum thyroxine level above normal are to be depreciated. There is an adverse effect on the heart and no benefit to the patient.

Other drugs have been used for the treatment of hypothyroidism but have little to commend them. Thyroid extract is prepared from the dried thyroid glands of animals. It is an impure substance of variable biological potency and a short shelf-life. It has now been deleted from the British National Formulary.

Triiodothyronine (T_3) is sometimes used but it has no advantages over thyroxine. Furthermore it produces at first sight some curious results in the tests used for assessing replacement therapy. By its action on the hypothalamus and the pituitary (Chapter 1), T_3 will suppress the secretion of TRH from the former and of TSH from the latter. Thus the TSH level will fall to normal when the correct dose of T_3 is being given. However the thyroid gland is incapable of making thyroxine and the administered T_3 will not be converted to T_4 so that the blood level of T_4 will remain abnormally low. Thus the only way of judging the correct dose of replacement T_3 is to measure the serum T_3 level and the technique for doing this is not universally available.

Hypothyroidism

Treatment of congenital and of juvenile hypothyroidism follows the same pattern as that for adult hypothyroidism although the optimal replacement dose of thyroxine will be smaller and will have to be increased as the baby or child grows. The initial dose for babies is 0.025 mg every day or every alternate day, and for children 0.05 mg daily. The correct dosage can best be determined by the serum thyroxine and TSH levels. Additional assessment of the response to treatment is made from the patient's growth in height and from the maturation of the bones as judged by a simple X-ray of the hand and wrist. Excessive dosage with thyroxine makes a patient of this age grow in height abnormally fast and become overactive and excitable.

8

Non-toxic goitre

The word 'goitre' means enlargement of the thyroid gland; 'non-toxic' means that the enlarged gland is not manufacturing an excess of the two thyroid hormones — T_4 and T_3 — and that the patient is euthyroid. It is often difficult in mild cases to decide whether the thyroid gland is enlarged beyond the upper limit of normal or not. The size varies from person to person, and it varies in different parts of the world, being larger in areas where there is iodine deficiency.

Causes of non-toxic goitre

There are many conditions and situations in which the thyroid gland becomes enlarged (Table 6).

Table 6 *Some common causes of non-toxic goitre*

Iodine deficiency (endemic goitre)
Hashimoto's autoimmune thyroiditis
Physiological or normal (puberty, pregnancy)
'Simple' non-toxic goitre
Foods and drugs that depress manufacture of thyroid hormones
Dyshormonogenesis (partial or complete failure of the thyroid cells to make thyroid hormones)
Cancer

Iodine deficiency is a well recognized cause of goitre. This occurs because of a lack of iodine in the diet and/or because the diet contains anti-thyroid or goitrogenic substances that prevent the thyroid from extracting iodine from the bloodstream or, if the iodine is trapped, prevent the thyroid cells from converting it to T_4 and T_3. World-wide iodine deficiency is the commonest cause of goitre. The iodine content of food, mainly sea fish, milk, and eggs, is largely dependent upon the fall of rain derived from sea-water. Thus iodine deficiency is found, or used to be found until corrective measures were taken, in areas far removed from the sea. Such was the case in Alpine countries such as Switzerland, around the Great Lakes in the United States, and even in the Pennines in England ('Derbyshire neck'). It is still common in large land-locked areas such as the Himalayas, in Iran, the Congo area, the Andes, and in New Guinea where preventative measures are imperfect. In these parts of the world goitre is so common that it effects 10 per cent or more of the population and is therefore called endemic.

In iodine-deficient regions there is a direct relationship between the degree of iodine deficiency and the prevalence of goitre. If the deficiency is marked, and this can be assessed by finding only very small amounts of iodine in a 24-hour urine collection, a large proportion of the population is likely to develop goitres. This is of importance to the public health authorities who can increase the iodine intake by adding iodide to the salt or flour which the population uses. In certain isolated areas such as New Guinea the incidence of goitre and the risk of an iodine-deficient goitrous mother giving birth to a hypothyroid baby has been reduced by giving every 3–5 years an intramuscular injection of iodized poppy-seed oil.

Hashimoto's thyroiditis as a cause of goitre is discussed in Chapter 6. It is in non-iodine-deficient areas of the world probably the most common cause for persistent thyroid enlargement.

Physiological goitre. Slight enlargement of the thyroid gland is common in girls at or soon after the onset of puberty. The reason for this is not known and the usual explanation given is that this is the time when the whole endocrine system is coming into full function.

Quite a number of women notice that their thyroid gland becomes slightly larger in the 10 to 7 days before their menstrual period.

Enlargement of the gland is common in pregnancy. In ancient Egypt it was the practice to tie a thin thread tightly round the neck of a young bride. When it broke she was known to be pregnant. Hormonal changes are in part responsible for the thyroid enlargement in pregnancy but a relative deficiency of iodine may arise. In a pregnant woman the growing fetus needs iodine and for unexplained reasons the woman excretes an increased amount of iodine in her urine during pregnancy; hence her body stores of iodine may become reduced unless her diet contains adequate amounts.

At the time of the menopause slight enlargement of the thyroid gland is not uncommon and may be looked upon as normal.

Simple non-toxic goitre. In this condition 'simple' has several meanings. It indicates both the normal secretory function of the gland and the absence of any malignant change within it. 'Simple' also implies that the cause of the goitre is unknown. In fact it would be clearer to both patient and doctor if it were called an idiopathic goitre — 'idiopathic' meaning of unknown origin. In fact the word 'simple' is something of a misnomer because finding the cause for a goitre may be far from simple nor is the treatment of it, if treatment is required at all, always simple either.

A simple non-toxic goitre may be smooth or nodular, symmetric or irregular in shape, small or large. Its cause is seldom discoverable. It is sometimes called a colloid goitre, a simple goitre, or a sporadic goitre (in contrast to the endemic goitre that occurs in iodine-deficient areas).

Foods and drugs, some recognized and many not, interfere with the trapping of iodine by the thyroid gland or with its conversion to T_4 and T_3. Cabbage, certain vegetables related to kale, and cassava have goitrogenic properties either when eaten by human beings or when human beings drink milk from cows that have been fed on kale. Certain medicines, notably cough and asthma cures, may cause thyroid enlargement when taken over a long time. Innumerable modern medicines, ranging from drugs used for the treatment of diabetes to those that cure tuberculosis, are goitrogenic to some degree with prolonged usage. A list would be extensive but in determining the cause of a goitre the doctor must be told precisely what drugs the patient is taking or has taken in the recent past.

Disturbed thyroid function (*dyshormonogenesis*). The making of T_4 and T_3 from its raw materials involves many orderly chemical steps, each of which is normally precisely regulated in just the same way as the manufacture of a car involves many distinct and supervised stages. A complete hold-up at any one stage will stop production of T_4 and T_3 and the patient would soon become hypothyroid. This seldom happens and more often there is a slowing up at one stage where production is inefficient. To compensate, the thyroid gland enlarges in the same way as when the production of cars slows at one point more men are put on in an attempt to circumvent the delaying inefficient process.

Disturbances of thyroid hormone synthesis may occur at any one of the many stages, and collectively this is called dyshormonogenesis which means literally 'disordered making of hormone'. To define the precise stage at which the hold-up is occurring requires specialized research techniques. Although of scientific interest, such knowledge may be of little practical benefit to the patient, because as yet we often do not know how actually to correct or improve the defective step. In most instances it is simpler to give the patient thyroxine by mouth and put the patient's thyroid gland to rest; this usually stops the goitre from getting larger and often makes it smaller. It also obviates the risk of the patient's becoming thyroid deficient.

Dyshormonogenic goitres tend to run in families. Usually the condition is apparent at or soon after birth because the baby has a small goitre. In other patients the abnormality does not become noticeable until after some years, because as the child grows and the need for thyroid hormone increases the gland enlarges in an attempt to meet the demand. In rare instances dyshormonogenesis is associated with other congenital defects such as deafness.

Cancer as a cause of goitre is discussed in Chapter 9.

Clinical picture of non-toxic goitre

Many people with a small but quite obvious non-toxic goitre are unaware of its presence and have no symptoms. A population study in England suggests that about 15 per cent of adults have a degree of thyroid enlargement, the prevalence being four times greater in women than men. Some patients become understandably apprehensive if they or a relative notice a fullness in the front of the neck, and fear they have cancer. It is therefore important to emphasize that cancer of the thyroid is extremely rare. Other patients on discovering a goitre immediately complain of 'a lump in the throat', difficulty in swallowing, or a choking feeling. Because large goitres seldom cause in many patients any symptoms at all, it is likely that the symptoms in those with a small goitre are more the consequence of apprehension than related to any thyroid enlargement. This applies particularly to those with a simple non-toxic goitre because some temporary discomfort is not uncommon in Hashimoto's thyroiditis (Chapter 6) and quite common in viral thyroiditis (Chapter 5). Sometimes a thyroid nodule or cyst is painful, particularly if a haemorrhage has occurred into it.

In many instances the investigation of patients with a non-toxic goitre is as important in allaying their fears as it is in trying to determine the cause of the thyroid enlargement and how best to treat it.

Thus the majority of non-toxic goitres produce no symptoms, and when these do occur they are best looked upon not as part and parcel of the usual clinical picture but as uncommon complications (see below).

What the doctor finds

Enlargement of the thyroid gland is initially slight. The gland may not even be visible when the chin is held high, but on feeling it the amount of thyroid tissue is greater than normal. Usually the enlargement effects the whole gland, which is uniformly and symmetrically increased in size and feels soft. If whatever is causing the goitre persists, further gradual enlargement of the gland may occur. First the gland is visible with the chin held high but later it may be seen with the head in a normal position. Over the years this enlargement may cease to be symmetrical so that one part of the gland becomes bigger than another. Thus one lobe may become more prominent than the other, or the isthmus may stand out more than the rest of the gland.

Sometimes smaller areas enlarge so that several nodules can be felt (a multinodular goitre). A fluid-containing cyst may develop in one of these nodules and cause a smooth rounded lump to appear (Plate 4). This is seldom painful or tender unless sudden bleeding occurs into the cyst. This may happen for no known reason; the smooth round swelling increases in size over a few hours, becomes hard because of the increased pressure inside it, and is very tender. If under local anaesthetic a needle is put into the lump, blood-stained fluid can be withdrawn; the lump becomes less tense and the pain is relieved.

Sometimes only one part of the one lobe becomes enlarged. This benign lump, called an adenoma, must be distinguished by the doctor from thyroid cancer (Chapter 9). Benign adenomas are much commoner than thyroid cancers; they seldom increase rapidly in size unless they become the site of an internal bleed; they are unattached to skin or deep structures and thus move freely with the rest of the gland on swallowing; and they take up technetium or radio-iodine normally as shown by an isotope scan.

Complications of a non-toxic goitre

Pressure symptoms. Left untreated a simple goitre may, rarely, grow to a considerable size, and by virtue of its mass cause local pressure symptoms. The large veins in the neck bringing blood back to the heart from the head may become compressed. The veins then stand out like thin ropes on one or both sides of the neck, and the patient may experience a sense of fullness in the head and face with the development of swelling just below the eyes and a general facial puffiness.

The windpipe may be compressed by a large goitre especially if the goitre or part of it lies low in the neck behind the sternum (p. 1). The windpipe may be pushed to one side and compressed by an asymmetrically enlarged gland. In extreme cases breathing is partially obstructed and on breathing out, particularly when asleep, the patient makes a crowing noise (stridor). This most often happens at night because when asleep the head may loll forward or to one side and the pressure on the windpipe increases.

Involvement of the nerves to the vocal cords. Very seldom indeed does pressure from a non-malignant goitre impair the function of the nerves to the vocal cords. Weakness or hoarseness of the voice suggests malignant invasion of one or both of the vocal cord nerves and calls for immediate investigation.

Hypothyroidism. Over the years a simple goitre may fail to provide sufficient T_4 and T_3 either because the initial cause of the goitre persists or because the gland becomes the site of autoimmune Hashimoto's thyroiditis (Chapter 6). Because of the possible development of hypothyroidism, patients with a goitre will often be asked to report to their doctor annually unless they are being treated with thyroxine which obviates any possibility of them becoming thyroid deficient.

Hyperthyroidism. The emergence of hyperthyroidism is less common. Occasionally an adenoma may cease to become responsive to the normal control exerted by TSH. The nodule becomes autonomous which means that it does not stop producing T_4 and T_3, as it should, when the TSH level falls. It has therefore become a toxic adenoma ('hot nodule' on isotope scanning) and the patient becomes thyrotoxic with all the symptoms and signs of hyperthyroidism (Chapter 4) except for the notable absence of important eye complications. The reason for the absence of ophthalmopathy is explained on p. 39.

Some patients with a multinodular goitre develop hyperthyroidism. In these an isotope scan may show increased activity in the cells between the nodules, and it is generally thought that the patient, who originally had just a multinodular goitre, has developed a second thyroid disorder, namely Graves' disease often with associated eye complications.

Diagnosis of non-toxic goitre

Although a careful history is taken and extensive tests may be made, it often proves impossible to determine the cause of a non-toxic goitre. Nevertheless it must be proved that the goitre is non-toxic and more importantly that there is no hypothyroidism or tendency to thyroid-hormone deficiency. A search for the cause of the goitre must be made but such a search need seldom go to the exhaustive lengths rightly pursued in a research laboratory. In essence the diagnosis of simple non-toxic goitre is made by proving a lot of negatives.

Thyroid disease: the facts

In simple non-toxic goitre there is no history of exposure to goitrogenic drugs or food and the T_4, T_3, and TSH levels are normal. When there is iodine deficiency, this may be suspected from the patient's geographical origin; she will probably know that she comes from an area of endemic goitre. A family history of goitre may suggest dyshormono-genesis and a mild form of this may well be the explanation for some idiopathic simple goitres. Either low levels of thyroid auto-antibodies or none at all will be present in the patient's serum. Isotope scans in the early stage of a goitre usually show a normal pattern of uniform uptake. With the development of multiple nodules, the uptake becomes patchy and irregular. Although a goitre may appear to contain on clinical examination a solitary nodule, thus suggesting the possibility of cancer (Chapter 9), often at surgery the gland is found to have multiple small nodules in it which cannot be felt from the outside. These may be detected by an isotope scan or an ultrasound scan and save the patient from having to have an exploratory operation.

The first evidence of liability to hypothyroidism, particularly in iodine deficiency, whether this is due to dietary lack or blockage of iodine uptake by thyroid cells due to a goitrogenic drug, is a low–normal or even abnormally low level of T_4 and a normal level of T_3. This occurs because the thyroid gland preferentially secretes T_3 under these circumstances rather than T_4 because this is more economical in the use of iodine; T_3 contains only three atoms of iodine as compared with the four iodine atoms in T_4. Later in the development of hypothyroidism, the T_4 will be below normal and the T_3 is normal but the TSH level is unequivocally raised. Eventually with the onset of clinical evidence of hypothyroidism, the TSH level rises further and the T_4 and T_3 both become abnormally low (Table 5, p. 68).

The uptake of radio-iodine or technetium given in a small tracer dose is normal in simple goitre. When there is iodine deficiency from dietary lack, the immediate uptake of the isotope is rapid and greater than normal because the starved thyroid tissue is avid for iodine. When a goitrogenic drug or foodstuff is blocking the uptake or utilization of iodine by the thyroid cells, the uptake of isotope will often also be blocked provided the goitrogenic substance is still being taken. As soon as the goitrogen is withdrawn and its effects have worn off, the isotope uptake is usually excessive because the thyroid tissue has been starved of iodine. In dyshormonogenic goitres the handling of radio-iodine or technetium varies depending on the particular stage impaired in the manufacture of hormone.

Treatment of non-toxic goitre

The logical approach to the treatment of any non-toxic goitre would be to correct or remove its cause. Because the cause of simple non-toxic goitre is not known, this is difficult. On the assumption that most cases are related either to slight, perhaps intermittent, iodine lack or to a minor degree of dyshormono-genesis or to both, control of the goitre is, however, usually possible.

First a normal dietary intake of iodine must be assured. Excess iodine, in the form of conventional doses of medicinal iodine (potassium iodide or Lugol's iodine) or 'health food' preparations such as kelp, may provide too much iodine and should usually be avoided. This is because in rare cases excess iodine induces hyperthyroidism, a condition known as the Jodd–Basedow phenomenon. The best source of dietary iodine is sea-salt or iodized salt. The former is available in many stores and health food shops, and the latter in most supermarkets where it is clearly labelled as 'iodized salt'. This type of salt should be used in cooking and at the table. Sea fish is a good source of iodine but expensive.

If the goitre is small and the patient is seen at a young age, an adequate intake of dietary iodine may be all that is necessary to prevent the gland from getting larger. Such treatment may make the goitre smaller, and it is wise to keep the patient under regular observation, initially every four months and later every 1-2 years for a few years. In the majority of instances nothing more is required.

If the gland increases in size with an adequate dietary intake of iodine or if the gland is large when the patient is first seen, treatment with thyroxine may be used. The initial dose may be 0.05 mg daily although this may be increased after a month to 0.1 mg daily. In patients aged from 15 to 25 this treatment is usually continued for about three years and then gradually reduced and finally stopped, a careful watch being kept on the size of the goitre. Thereafter in some patients the position remains static; in others the thyroid begins to enlarge again and lifelong thyroxine treatment with regular supervision is necessary.

Some patients may fail to seek advice until too late. By this time the enlarged thyroid may be cosmetically unsightly; it may be a multinodular goitre or it may contain a sizeable adenoma. In these cases subtotal thyroidectomy may have to be considered and surgical treatment will certainly be indicated if the goitre is causing compression symptoms and will also probably be required if the gland is retrosternal. In almost every patient after surgery thyroxine treatment (see Chapter 7) will be required to prevent recurring enlargement of the remaining thyroid tissue.

9

Cancer of the thyroid gland

Compared with the incidence of malignancy elsewhere in the body, cancer of the thyroid gland is rare, constituting less than 0.5 per cent of all deaths from malignant diseases. Although it may occur at any age, it is most common between the ages of 30 and 60, and as with other thyroid disorders there is a preponderance of women.

Although the precise cause is unknown, two separate factors appear to predispose to the development of thyroid cancer. The first is undue exposure to X-ray radiation of the head, neck, or chest. There was a vogue in the 1930s, particularly in certain centres in the United States of America, to reduce the size of enlarged tonsils and adenoids in children by X-ray therapy in preference to surgical removal. A significant number of children treated in this way have developed thyroid cancer 10–40 years later. Similarly the treatment by X-rays of red birth-marks on the face or neck of infants may later give rise to cancer of the thyroid gland. In Japan survivors of the atomic bomb have since the late 1950s shown an increase in malignant thyroid nodules.

The second factor is a pre-existing goitre which, irrespective of its cause, seems to increase slightly the risk of malignant change developing. This however is rare and an uncommon association. Only about 350 patients (6 per million of the population) die each year in England and Wales of thyroid cancer, but any sudden change in the shape of a pre-existing goitre or the development of discomfort or pain calls for careful investigation.

Types of thyroid cancer

Thyroid cancers can be separated into two main groups — differentiated and undifferentiated or anaplastic.

Differentiated cancers. In these the cells that have become malignant continue to look like normal thyroid cells and behave like normal thyroid cells in that they may continue to respond to the stimulating action of TSH and to take up iodine from the bloodstream. These differentiated cancers are divided into follicular and papillary sub-groups according to the pattern in which the cells arrange themselves — a pattern that may be difficult to distinguish under the microscope from normal thyroid tissue. These tumours are relatively 'civilized'; they grow slowly and spread to distant parts of the body late. The fact that they often continue to take up radio-iodine makes the detection of secondary deposits or metastases (the spread of the tumour to other parts of the body) easier and allows effective treatment to be given by irradiating the metastases with radio-iodine. Also if the secretion of TSH from the pituitary is reduced to negligible amounts by giving thyroxine by mouth, the stimulus for the cancer cells to grow is diminished.

Undifferentiated cancers. Less commonly the cells of thyroid cancer are undifferentiated. These 'uncivilized' anaplastic cells, like anarchists, are uncontrolled and uncontrollable. They multiply rapidly and invade surrounding structures in the neck, which often makes surgical removal impossible.

Medullary-cell cancer. A very rare form of thyroid cancer may develop from cells which are not strictly speaking thyroid cells at all but 'lodgers' living in the thyroid gland. These so-called 'C-cells' or para-follicular or medullary cells do not secrete T_4 or T_3. They manufacture a hormone known as calcitonin (hence 'C-cells') which regulates the amount of calcium in the bones. They may secrete other hormones which increase the activity of the intestines and hence

92

Cancer of the thyroid gland

induce diarrhoea. These rare medullary-cell cancers tend to run in families and to be associated with small non-malignant tumours in the abdomen (phaeochromocytomas) that secrete excess adrenaline (epinephrine) and noradrenaline (norepinephrine), hormones that cause high blood pressure. Because so rare, medullary-cell cancers will not be considered further except to say that surgical removal both of the malignant medullary-cell tumour in the neck and the associated benign phaeochromocytoma(s) in the abdomen is often successful.

Lymphomas. Sometimes the thyroid is the site of a malignant lymphoma, a tumour arising from lymphocytes or related cells residing in the thyroid gland. Lymphomas are often fast growing so that the thyroid increases rapidly in size and may compress the windpipe to cause shortness of breath or a crowing noise (stridor) when the patient breathes out. These tumours are usually sensitive to X-ray therapy.

Metastatic cancer. The thyroid occasionally becomes the site of secondary deposits from cancer of the lung, breast, or kidney, but at this stage the primary growth will usually have declared itself.

Clinical picture of thyroid cancer

In the most common types of differentiated cancer (follicular or papillary) the initial manifestation is usually the development of a small lump in the thyroid gland. This lump is round and nodular, often hard to the touch, usually but not always painless, and may initially be no bigger than a pea. The thyroid gland may formerly have been perfectly normal or it may have been enlarged for many years.

Sometimes more than one lump develops, because these differentiated cancers tend to be multifocal in origin; that is to say they start in different parts of the gland at the same time. The malignant cells may spread to neighbouring lymph nodes in the neck. The patient may then present with a 'swollen gland' which is an enlarged painless lymph node, and little or nothing to suggest that the primary growth is in the thyroid gland itself.

Left untreated differentiated thyroid cancer will spread (metastasize) to other parts of the body, the malignant cells being carried in the bloodstream or the lymphatic system to the lungs, the liver, or the bones. Not until there has been considerable destruction of a bone by a metastasis does the patient feel pain, and this pain may occur suddenly if the bone breaks without any preceding fall or unusual force being applied (a 'pathological fracture').

An undifferentiated anaplastic type of thyroid cancer tends to occur in older patients. The gland enlarges and becomes generally tender. The highly malignant cells may invade the overlying skin, making it red as though there were acute inflammation. Deeper structures in the neck may be invaded so that on swallowing the gland does not move up and down in the neck as freely as it should. Involvement of the nerves to the vocal cords makes the patient's voice weak or husky, and this may occur with any type of thyroid cancer.

Diagnosis of thyroid cancer

The diagnosis is made on the basis of clinical suspicion and confirmed by biopsy. Clinical suspicion will be aroused if there is sudden enlargement in a pre-existing goitre, a previous history of exposure of the upper part of the body to X-rays, pain in the thyroid gland in the absence of evidence of auto-immune or viral thyroiditis, hoarseness or weakness of the voice, or the development of an asymmetrical lump or a nodule in a previously normal thyroid gland.

Isotope scanning using technetium or radio-iodine, or first one and then the other, may be helpful in deciding that cancer is probably not present but is less helpful in confirming that it is. Although malignant cells may take up technetium, they seldom do so as avidly as surrounding normal thyroid cells. Thus the technetium scan may show that the area under suspicion is 'cold' or relatively 'cold' as compared with the neighbouring normal thyroid tissue. Even if the uptake of technetium appears normal, a radio-iodine scan should be done to confirm that not only have the cells the ability to trap iodine (i.e. extract iodine from the bloodstream) but that they are also capable of converting the trapped iodine into T_4 and T_3.

Thus if the technetium and the radio-iodine scans are both normal, it is most improbable that the tissue is malignant. If on the other hand the technetium scan is normal, signifying that the cells in the area can extract iodine from the bloodstream, but the radio-iodine scan is abnormal, indicating that the synthesis of T_4 and T_3 is defective, the tissue may be malignant and should be subjected to biopsy.

If the tissue under suspicion does not take up technetium, it may be malignant although other conditions, such as a benign cyst or an area of autoimmune or viral thyroiditis, may produce a similar 'cold' spot on the scan. If the area is 'cold', a biopsy should be done.

When a biopsy is required, an open surgical procedure is preferred. While the patient is still anaesthetized, the tissue under suspicion can be examined under the microscope by quickly freezing the cells and when they are frozen solid cutting the tissue into thin slices (a 'frozen section'). If the microscopical appearance is that of cancer, a careful search is made for other malignant foci in the same and in the other lobe of the thyroid gland. If no further malignancy is found, the lobe on the affected side is removed but as there is often doubt as to the normality of the rest of the gland, many surgeons recommend complete removal of all thyroid tissue (a total thyroidectomy).

Tests of thyroid secretory function, the T_4 and T_3 levels, should be done but are seldom helpful in the diagnosis of thyroid cancer. Only very rarely indeed is a thyroid cancer the cause of thyrotoxicosis. Thyroid autoantibodies should be looked for. Their presence does not exclude cancer, but the higher the level the more likely is autoimmune thyroiditis as opposed to malignancy.

An enlarged cervical lymph node. There are many trivial and serious causes for an enlarged lymph node on one side of the neck, ranging from a simple infection or glandular fever (infective mononucleosis) to tuberculosis and cancer. Clinical examination and relatively simple investigations will usually establish the cause. In obscure diagnostic cases an isotope scan may show that technetium is taken up by the node. This strongly suggests that the lymph node is the site of metastatic spread from a hidden primary tumour in the thyroid gland, and surgical removal must be planned accordingly.

 Treatment of thyroid cancer

An anaplastic cancer of the thyroid is best treated by deep X-ray therapy though in its earliest stages surgical removal followed by X-ray therapy may be possible.

The treatment of a differentiated-cell thyroid cancer is a great deal more satisfactory. At the initial surgical operation not only is the malignant area removed and also neighbouring lymph nodes which may be the site of early metastases but usually also the rest of the seemingly normal gland. This is done because of the possibility that other small malignant foci may be present in the apparently normal gland and because total thyroidectomy makes subsequent management of the patient easier and more effective. In skilled hands total thyroidectomy can usually be accomplished without damage to the nerves to the vocal cords and without loss of all the parathyroid glands with resultant tetany (Chapter 4, p. 51).

When the patient has recovered from the operation, a large ablative therapeutic dose of radio-iodine is given with the objective of destroying any residual thyroid cells, normal or malignant, although the normal cells will usually take up more of the radio-iodine than the malignant ones. Replacement

Cancer of the thyroid gland

therapy with thyroxine or triiodothyronine is started in a dose which keeps the blood T_4 or T_3 level in the upper half of the normal range and which also, and this is important, suppresses the secretion of TSH. By keeping the TSH at a low level any remaining malignant thyroid cells are not exposed to its stimulating action and may remain dormant.

After six months it is common practice to withdraw the substitution therapy. After 2–4 weeks off replacement treatment, when the TSH level has risen to 20 mU/l or higher, a small tracer dose of radio-iodine is given. An isotope scan of the neck and of the whole body is then done. If any significant number of thyroid cells, normal or malignant, remain in the neck they will show up on the scan and so also will any significant number of differentiated malignant cells that have formed secondary deposits elsewhere in the body. If the scans show evidence of residual thyroid tissue that takes up radio-iodine a further large therapeutic dose of radio-iodine is given and the replacement treatment started again. This procedure is repeated annually so that any recurrence of the cancer can be detected and treated. Although the outcome is generally satisfactory, this method of assessing recurrence is expensive because of the neck and whole-body scans involved and has the theoretical disadvantage that any residual malignant cells are exposed for a time to the stimulating effect of high TSH levels when the maintenance therapy is temporarily stopped.

In future it may prove unnecessary to follow this technique. It has been found that the level of thyroglobulin (Chapter 1, p. 4), which is present in small amounts in the bloodstream of normal subjects, is increased in patients with differentiated thyroid cancers even when they are receiving replacement therapy. Thus measurement of the blood thyroglobulin level may prove an effective indicator of the presence or absence of *residual* thyroid cancer and only when the level becomes abnormally high need isotope studies be made and further radio-iodine treatment given.

10

Miscellaneous disorders of the thyroid gland

A number of miscellaneous disorders of the thyroid gland, not dealt with elsewhere in this book or in need of special consideration, are discussed in this chapter.

Pituitary disease and the thyroid

Although the relationship between the pituitary gland, TSH, and the thyroid gland has been discussed in Chapter 1, little mention has been made of the thyroid disorders that may develop as a secondary consequence of pituitary disease.

Very rarely indeed does overactivity of the thyroid gland result from increased secretion of TSH by the pituitary (p. 34).

Failure of the pituitary gland to secrete TSH is more common and causes secondary thyroid failure. The resulting deficiency in the secretion of thyroid hormones induces a clinical picture very similar to the hypothyroidism that follows primary thyroid failure (Chapter 7). This picture is often modified, however, by additional features which are the consequence of alterations in the secretion of the several other pituitary hormones that influence growth, sexual development and function, and adrenal gland activity.

Reduced production of TSH is usually due to a tumour destroying the pituitary gland. In addition to failure of the distant thyroid and other target glands (Chapter 1, p. 3), the tumour may cause local symptoms in the skull, such as headaches and disturbances of vision.

Treatment involves dealing with the pituitary tumour itself and giving replacement therapy not only to make good the deficiency of the thyroid gland but also for that of the other

Miscellaneous disorders of the thyroid gland

glands, the ovaries or testes and the adrenal glands, which may have become underactive too.

Pregnancy and the thyroid

The regulatory role of the thyroid gland in controlling metabolism is at no time less important than in pregnancy.

Women with either hyperthyroidism or thyroid deficiency tend to have difficulty in conceiving but this relative infertility is reversible. Many hyperthyroid patients quickly become pregnant as soon as their hyperthyroidism is controlled with an antithyroid drug such as carbimazole or methimazole. Heavy menstrual loss in hypothyroid women is often corrected by replacement therapy with thyroxine, normal menstrual cycles with regular ovulation resume, and pregnancy occurs.

Normal pregnancy. In normal pregnancy the thyroid gland often enlarges (p. 82). This is in part due to a minor degree of iodine deficiency which develops because of the fetal demands for iodine and the increased excretion of iodine in the mother's urine. In part the thyroid enlargement may also be due to certain hormones formed in the placenta. The slight enlargement of the mother's thyroid is of no consequence but she should ensure an adequate dietary intake of iodine by using sea-salt or iodized salt in the kitchen and at the table and having sea-fish at least once weekly.

Pregnancy in a hypothyroid woman. It is most important that a hypothyroid woman taking replacement therapy with thyroxine, which therefore is keeping her euthyroid, should continue taking the same dose of thyroxine throughout her pregnancy, delivery, and thereafter.

Confusion may arise because in a normal pregnant woman and also in a hypothyroid woman taking a constant replacement dose of thyroxine the total serum thyroxine level increases in pregnancy. The rise in serum T_4 may be quite substantial because the amount of carrier-protein or thyroxine-binding protein normally increases during pregnancy. Thus a woman, taking a constant dose of T_4, which gave her a normal total T_4 blood level before she became pregnant, may be found to have a higher than normal level during pregnancy. Unless the reason for this is understood there will be an obvious temptation to reduce the dose of replacement T_4, which is uncalled for.

Pregnancy in a thyrotoxic woman. This is best avoided by rendering the patient euthyroid before she becomes pregnant and ensuring that she remains euthyroid. In most instances the hyperthyroidism is therefore best treated, after appropriate preparation, by subtotal thyroidectomy before conception takes place.

If hyperthyroidism occurs in pregnancy, either because the patient has been treated in the past with antithyroid drugs and has now relapsed or because the thyrotoxicosis has developed *de novo*, two forms of treatment may be used. Either a subtotal thyroidectomy, after due preparation, can be done during the second trimester with little risk to the mother or fetus and little danger of provoking a miscarriage, or the mother can be treated with an antithyroid drug such as carbimazole with or without propranolol. The minimal effective dose of carbimazole or methimazole should be used, because these compounds cross the placenta. Treatment with antithyroid drugs should be stopped, except in particularly florid cases, some 4–6 weeks before delivery. In most instances the fetus is not adversely effected although sometimes the baby is born with a small goitre which disappears spontaneously.

Lactating mothers taking carbimazole or methimazole may secrete the drug in their milk, and it is generally advised that they should not breast-feed. There is now some doubt as to whether sufficient carbimazole or methimazole is secreted in the milk to effect the baby, but this is a problem currently being looked into.

Miscellaneous disorders of the thyroid gland

Neonatal hyperthyroidism. Congenital hyperthyroidism in a new-born infant is very rare. It occurs only in an infant born of a mother who currently has Graves' disease or has in the past been treated for Graves' disease. The cause lies in the thyroid-stimulating antibodies that have induced the Graves' disease in the mother, and which may persist after she has been rendered euthyroid and then cross the placenta to induce overactivity of the thyroid gland of the fetus.

Very few babies of previously thyrotoxic mothers are in fact effected, but are more likely to be so if the mother has severe eye complications of Graves' disease or pretibial myxoedema (p. 37) — both findings which suggest continuation of high maternal thyroid-stimulating antibody levels.

In such women the possibility of the baby's being thyrotoxic should be considered during the later part of pregnancy. Intra-uterine fetal hyperthyroidism may be suspected if the fetal heart-rate is unduly fast and if there is abnormal fetal growth as judged by an ultrasound scan, which can, without any damage to the baby, measure fetal development. If there is evidence of intra-uterine thyrotoxicosis, the fetal overactive thyroid gland can be controlled by giving the mother carbimazole or methimazole, which crosses the placenta and will damp down the fetal thyroid gland. During this treatment any possibility of the mother's becoming hypothyroid can be obviated by giving her in addition thyroxine which barely crosses the placental barrier and thus will not effect the fetus.

If a baby is born with neonatal hyperthyroidism it usually has slight enlargement of the thyroid gland. The heart-rate is unduly rapid and the baby is restless. Minimal eye signs may be present but the main feature is the failure of the baby to thrive and it may have diarrhoea. The diagnosis is confirmed by finding a raised serum thyroxine level.

Treatment must be given urgently with small doses of iodine (Lugol's iodine, p. 45) and carbimazole in half the adult amount. Fortunately the neonatal hyperthyroidism is self-limiting, because the thyroid-stimulating antibodies from the mother persist in the new-born baby for only three months. Thus active treatment is required for only this period of time.

Maternal Hashimoto's thyroiditis. Mothers with Hashimoto's autoimmune thyroiditis and normal thyroid function seldom experience any particular difficulty during pregnancy. After delivery however there is a tendency, often only temporary, for the autoimmune thyroiditis to worsen. This may lead in the postpartum period to the mother becoming overtly hypothyroid. Treatment with thyroxine will be required and this may be necessary for only a few months or permanently.

Hyperthyroid crisis

This is, or used to be, a rare complication of hyperthyroidism and usually occurred, in the past, in patients with Graves' disease who were operated upon without proper preparation. Occasionally it occurred in untreated hyperthyroid patients who developed an intercurrent infection such as influenza, a streptococcal sore throat, or pneumonia. In the old days before there were antithyroid drugs such as carbimazole or methimazole, the patient was given only Lugol's iodine pre-operatively (p. 45). This was adequate if the surgeon ensured that the patient had become euthyroid as judged by slowing of the pulse rate (particularly the sleeping pulse), a gain in weight, and a substantial lessening of the symptoms and other signs of hyperthyroidism. It was common practice to avoid thyroid surgery during the hot summer months. Nowadays proper pre-operative preparation of the patient is attained with antithyroid drugs and a beta-blocker, such as propranolol; and thyrotoxicosis does not go unrecognized or untreated.

Because patients and surgeons may be in a hurry to achieve a cure, there is in my view, and not mine alone, an unfortunate practice today for subtotal thyroidectomy to be carried out in patients prepared for operation solely with propranolol. Certainly propranolol may bring substantial improvements in

102

the symptoms and signs of thyrotoxicosis but it does not render the patient biochemically euthyroid. In most such instances the patient (and the surgeon) get away with it without the development of a post-operative thyroid crisis but this is not a universally safe practice.

A thyroid crisis or storm, as it used to be called, is characterized by a relatively sudden and severe exacerbation of thyrotoxicosis. The patient develops a fever, a very rapid pulse rate often associated with irregularity of the heart-beat (atrial fibrillation), profound sweating with loss of body water, a state of shock with a low blood pressure, and mental confusion or delirium. The outcome may be fatal.

The condition is due to the release of an excess of thyroid hormones into the bloodstream as the surgeon handles the incompletely prepared thyroid gland during its subtotal removal. More conventional pre-operative treatment prevents this happening.

Apathetic hyperthyroidism

This is a rare, and rather mysterious, condition that seems to occur only in older patients with neglected, undiagnosed, and untreated thyrotoxicosis. The clinical picture is such that the diagnosis of apathetic hyperthyroidism may easily escape recognition because it is divergent from that seen in ordinary thyrotoxicosis.

The patient is depressed and emotionally flat. This is in marked contrast to the usual picture of anxiety and emotional over-alertness. Instead of being restless the patient is lethargic and underactive. Although there may be a history or evidence of weight loss, the patient appears bloated.

In a sophisticated medical community apathetic hyperthyroidism is extremely rare. It responds to antithyroid drug treatment.

The solitary 'cold' nodule

The development of what appears to be a solitary or single nodule in the thyroid gland is not uncommon and often gives rise to concern because of the possibility that the nodule might be an early cancer. In many instances the nodule is first noticed by a friend or relative of the patient or is found by a doctor on routine examination. Thyroid cancer is uncommon and in most cases the fear of malignancy proves ill-founded.

If the nodule on isotope scanning takes up technetium and therefore has the ability to trap iodine it is probably not malignant. If it also takes up radio-iodine it is definitely not malignant.

The problem is more difficult if the nodule is 'cold' and does not take up technetium. Although a cancer may be the cause of the nodule there are other more common possibilities. (1) The nodule may in fact be an innocent cyst, and identifiable as such by an ultrasound scan (p. 85). (2) The nodule may be a localized area of autoimmune thyroiditis but this is less easy to be sure of even if there are quite high levels of thyroid antibodies in the patient's blood. (3) Quite often what feels like a solitary nodule proves at operation to be a large nodule in a thyroid gland that contains many other smaller nodules that cannot be felt through the skin.

Often it is impossible to be certain of the nature of a 'cold' nodule without removing it at a surgical biopsy, although sometimes a needle or drill biopsy (p. 28) provides the diagnosis. Whenever there is any doubt, and particularly if the patient is a child or an adult under the age of 40 without any pre-existing goitre, surgical removal is the wisest course. This may be alarming to the patient but the diagnosis must not be less than one hundred per cent certain and if an early cancer is found the outlook is very good indeed.

Miscellaneous disorders of the thyroid gland

Riedel's thyroiditis

This is an extremely rare condition in which the thyroid becomes replaced by scarring fibrous tissue. The gland feels as hard as wood ('ligneous thyroiditis'). It becomes attached to the overlying skin and to deeper structures so that the windpipe is constricted and involvement of the nerves to the vocal cords causes hoarseness or weakness of the voice. Swallowing may be difficult. Without an open surgical biopsy it is seldom possible to distinguish this condition from an anaplastic cancer of the thyroid gland (p. 92), and an operation is usually required to relieve the constriction of the trachea.

Reidel's thyroiditis may be associated with a similar fibrosis affecting the covering of the intestines (peritoneal fibrosis), structures at the back of the abdomen (retroperitoneal fibrosis) so that the flow of urine down the tubes (the ureters) from the kidneys to the bladder is impeded, the duct that carries bile from the liver to the intestines (sclerosing cholangitis) resulting in jaundice, and structures in the centre of the thorax (mediastinal fibrosis). The cause of this very uncommon condition is unknown.

Suppurative thyroiditis

Rarely the thyroid gland is infected by pus-forming micro-organisms such as staphylococci which are the cause of boils. Other infections of the gland may be due to streptococci, tubercle bacilli, or syphilis. In these rare infections involving the thyroid gland, the picture may be dominated by more widespread infection in other parts of the body. The response to an appropriate antibiotic is usually rapid.

105

11

Epilogue

Medicine is not an exact science; probably it never will be because no two patients are ever the same. Their susceptibility and their physical, biological, and psychological reactions to the same disease will always differ. Equally doctors are likely to vary somewhat in their management of a patient's illness. No one course of action or treatment is necessarily more 'right' than another.

Patients, or the relatives and friends of patients, may be concerned that the treatment prescribed may not always follow closely the practices advocated in this book, practices which are the synthesis of the experience of just one doctor. Apparent minor differences should not disturb them because the basic scientific principles are widely accepted. Nevertheless the details of management may vary form one centre to another depending upon differences in the population being treated, the availability of technical facilities, laboratory expertise, and financial considerations.

In the treatment of thyroid diseases the art of managing the special needs and idiosyncrasies of a particular patient may contribute as much to the outcome as the science.

Glossary of drugs

Throughout the text the 'common' name has been used for each drug mentioned. These 'common' names are likely to be familiar to doctors world-wide. Some doctors prescribe drugs of a particular proprietary brand and this may be confusing to the patient, who may not know the contents of the proprietary tablet.

Below is given a short glossary of the drugs most often used in the treatment of patients with thyroid disorders. In each instance the drug is first identified by its 'common' name. Then its official name, as it appears in a pharmacopoeia, is given. This is followed by a list of proprietary names, a list which cannot be all-inclusive because different brand names are used in different countries and in different marketing areas throughout the world. Finally a brief indication is given of the purpose for which the drug is usually used in patients with thyroid disease.

Thyroxine (T_4)

Official names: levothyroxine sodium, L-thyroxine sodium, levothyroxinum natricum, thyroxine sodium.

Proprietary names: Cytoden, Eltroxin, Euthyrox, Letter, Levaxin, Levoid, Oroxine, Percutacrine thyroxinique, Synthroid, Thyratabs, Thyroxevan, Thyrine, Thyroxinal.

Use: As replacement therapy in deficiency of thyroid hormone.

Tri-iodothyronine (T_3)

Official names: liothyronine sodium, liothyroninum natricum, L-triiodothyronine, sodium liothyronine, triiodothyronine sodium.

Proprietary names: Cynomel, Cytomel, Tertroxin, Triacana, Trithyrone.

Use: As replacement therapy in deficiency of thyroid hormone.

Mixtures of thyroxine and triiodothyronine

Official names: none.

Proprietary names: Liotrix (contains thyroxine and triiodothyronine in a 4:1 ratio). Dithyron (thyroxine 0.05 mg and triiodothyronine 12.5 µg)

Glossary

Use: As a replacement therapy in deficiency of thyroid hormones.

Thyroglobulin

Official name: thyroglobulin.

Proprietary name: Proloid.

Use: As replacement therapy in deficiency of thyroid hormone.

Thyroid extract

Official names: dry thyroid, Getrocknete Schilddrüse, thyroid extract, thyreoidin, thyroidea, thyroideum sicca, tiroide secca.

Proprietary names: S-P-T, Thyranon, Thyrar, Thyroboline, Thyrocrine.

Use: As replacement therapy in deficiency of thyroid hormone.

Carbimazole

Official names: carbimazole, carbimazolum.

Proprietary names: Carbazole, Neo-mercazole, Neo-morphazole, Neo-thyreostat, Thyrostat.

Use: For control or treatment of hyperthyroidism.

Methimazole

Official names: methimazole, mercazolylum, thiamazolum.

Proprietary names: Favistan, Tapazole, Thacapzol.

Use: For control or treatment of hyperthyroidism.

Propylthiouracil

Official names: propylthiouracil, propylthiouracilum.

Proprietary names: Propycil, Propyl-thyracil, Thyreostat II, Tiotil.

Use: For control or treatment of hyperthyroidism.

Thyrotrophin-releasing hormone (TRH)

Official names: lopremone, protirelin, thyroliberin, thyrotrophin-releasing hormone, TRH.

Use: For the special investigation of thyroid gland function.

Glossary

Propranolol

Official names: propranolol, propranolol hydrochloride.

Proprietary names: Aviocardyl, Berkolol, Dociton, Herzul, Inderal, Inderalici, Kemi, Sumial.

Index

Index

Index